Why is American Healthcare so Expensive?

Solving the Puzzle of American Healthcare Costs to Build a Low-Cost System

Harvey Singh, Ph.D.

Why is American Healthcare so Expensive?

Solving the Puzzle of American Healthcare Costs to Build a Low-Cost System

Printed in the United States of America

Library of Congress

IISBN-13: 978-1519771797

ISBN-10: 1519771797

Dedication

These pages are dedicated to all Americans who would like to live healthy lives but who do not have the money to spend on U.S. healthcare.

Disclaimer

The content of this publication is for informational purposes. Any ideas and suggestions pertaining to your health in this book are not intended as a substitute for consulting with your physician or healthcare practitioner.

Why This Book?

This book will be of interest to anyone who is frustrated with the ever-rising costs of American medicine and wants to take a behind-the-scenes look at what is causing this trend.

Written for the layperson and the expert alike, it explains why our healthcare market in which the providers depend heavily upon insurance companies for payments is not a free market. Add to that the practice of paying doctors on a fee-for-service basis, and we have created a market with perverse incentives for nearly all the market players.

This has resulted in a system of care in which medical mistakes are ubiquitous, malpractice lawsuits are common, and 'end of life' medical costs are astronomical. In fact, medicine has become more dangerous than the disease and a single look at the price tag for some of the treatments can trigger a heart attack.

But these seemingly diverse and apparently unrelated problems have common origins. The book identifies the common elements at the root of these problems. Then it goes on to show how most problems can be solved by fundamentally changing the way we deliver medicine to our citizens.

TABLE OF CONTENTS

ACKNOWLEDGMENTS

I am grateful to Steven Stauffer for diligently editing the manuscript in its earlier stages and providing encouragement by offering valuable criticism and comments. Without his help, this book would not have been possible. Thanks are also due to Allison Bell who offered valuable advice for enhancing the readability and quality of the content. I am also grateful to Alice Heiserman who helped put everything together in the final stages of publication and made the publication of this book eventually possible.

Thanks are due to my wife, Kustantina, for supporting me through this lengthy project and making sacrifices in our day-to-day life to help get the project completed.

Last but not the least, I would like to acknowledge many others in my life who I could not acknowledge earlier yet their influence in my life has been critical. I want to thank the faculty and staff at the University of Oklahoma who guided me during my graduate studies at the University. I would especially like to thank Dr. Jon G Bredeson, my thesis advisor, whose influence I feel to this day as I continue to be inspired by it.

If, as a nation, we try to solve problems that are the result of high healthcare costs without trying to understand the underlying reasons that are driving up the prices, it would be like trying to get rid of the symptoms of a disease without understanding its origins.

INTRODUCTION

American healthcare costs have reached perilous levels. They are wreaking havoc not only on individual Americans but on our nation as a whole. Thousands of Americans are suffering because they cannot afford healthcare. Many more lose all their possessions and have to declare bankruptcies just because they were unlucky and got sick. Our Social Security system is also being threatened because rising healthcare costs put the retirement of millions of Americans at risk.

That is not all. American corporations, too, have trouble competing abroad because of the high healthcare premiums that they must pay for their employees. This decreases our nation's competitiveness and eventually may lower the American standard of living. Like cancer, the American healthcare system threatens to consume even the previously healthy sectors of the economy.

Although the sky-rocketing costs are an acute problem, few Americans understand the reasons behind what makes American medicine ominously expensive. Not even many policymakers comprehend the reasons behind the unrestrained growth of these expenses.

If, as a nation, we try to solve problems that are the result of high costs without trying to understand the underlying reasons that are driving up the prices, it would be like trying to get rid

1

of the symptoms of a disease without understanding its origins. For this reason, despite so many reforms by many presidents, our nation is still struggling to find satisfactory solutions.

President Lyndon B. Johnson enacted Medicare and Medicaid. Although these programs helped provide healthcare to the elderly and the poor, they left the cost problem untouched. His programs may have inadvertently contributed to accelerating medical costs; thus, making it more expensive for future generations. Similarly, President Bill Clinton's Children's Health Insurance Program (CHIP) extended healthcare access to children. This also occurred without changing the system to bring down costs.

As of this writing, President Barack Obama's *Patient Protection and Affordable Care Act* (ACA), also known as "Obamacare," is being implemented. This landmark law makes a serious attempt to provide universal coverage to U.S citizens.[1] For the first time in the U.S history, all Americans will be guaranteed the opportunity to buy health insurance regardless of their health or financial status. But, this law suffers from same shortcomings as the previous laws.

Although the ACA legislation takes steps to put more accountability and more efficiency into the system, it appears to have failed in controlling the price of healthcare. The provisions for cost and quality control have not been able to slow down the rise in *overall* costs, nor do they promise to lower the costs in the future because the law does not address the core problem with our healthcare system: what is causing the runaway rising medical costs in the first place.

After all, it is the rising costs that have been responsible for significant numbers of people becoming uninsured. By not paying attention to how the law might impact future costs, it could worsen the problem for future generations.

Some unintended consequences occurred following the implementation of the ACA. American businesses have started to drop people from their payrolls to get around the provisions of this act. So, a law that was enacted with good intentions could end up exasperating the problems that it was intended to solve.

Present day healthcare costs are not the only problem. A worrisome aspect is the pattern of *growth of medical expenditures over the last few decades*. The Centers for Medicare and Medicaid Services (CMS) have calculated the national healthcare spending over the last several years.[2] Using this data to plot the costs on a graph, the resulting curve has a hockey-stick shape. That is, not only are the healthcare costs rising but their rate of growth has also been increasing.

Until we can understand and curb the factors that are responsible for the shape of the cost-curve, future spending can be expected to follow the same pattern as in the past. If we cannot change the shape of this curve, we have failed to find a long-term solution for controlling costs.

So what is at the heart of the American Healthcare problem?

This book will show that at the root of most of our problems is our *incorrect belief that our healthcare is based on a free-market system*. Much of our present inability to understand or fix the problems stems from this false belief. This is also the reason our system is full of paradoxes that arise directly or indirectly from the belief that we have a free-market system. Since free markets produce excellent results in most areas of economy, many believe that we already have the best possible system that we can hope for, and it should not be changed.

But, some readers might have observed that our system is producing results that are opposite to those found in free markets. Despite being the most expensive system in the world, the American system is rated near the bottom in most categories among all the industrialized nations.[3] The United States ranks thirty-first out of thirty-four Organization for Economic Cooperation and Development (OECD) countries for infant mortality.[4] The Commonwealth Fund recently rated the United States dead last in healthcare rankings among the eleven industrialized countries it studied.[5]

Some legislators also mistakenly believe we have free markets in healthcare. They have suggested reforms based on that assumption. But, the reforms that can work well in free-markets will not work in a system such as ours.

Of course, the biggest victims of the convoluted healthcare markets are the American people. The issue is creating a rift between the 'haves' and the 'have-nots.' The 'haves,' who oppose universal coverage, seem to be opposing it because of misunderstandings and false beliefs.

First, they believe that universal coverage will *necessarily* mean more taxes. They are not aware that everyone can be covered without imposing more taxes if the costs of healthcare are brought down to reasonable levels. Second, some upper middle class Americans believe that just because they can afford healthcare *today*, they are not vulnerable in the *future*. What they might not realize is that sickness can severely limit their earning abilities in the future so that rapidly accelerating costs could put them at risk too.

Today's medical prices are so outrageous that even after being insured, some people have to declare bankruptcy because they are unable to pay even the insurance *deductibles*. Even those receiving a subsidy under the *Affordable Care Act*, might find it difficult to pay the deductibles—especially when their earning powers are reduced due to sickness. Even wealthy Americans are vulnerable in our system and can lose their property if catastrophic illness strikes.

Besides these problems, our country is burdened with the 'end of life' cost-problem.[6] Many people routinely lose most of their lifetime savings to medical expenses toward the end of their lives. Despite working hard, many die destitute. Some people have accepted this phenomenon as inevitable, and do not realize that there is no basic reason for this to occur. There is no reason why a catastrophic illness must wipe out one's lifetime savings. The only reason it is happening in our country is because of a badly designed healthcare system.

We *can* lower the costs by changing the system. The changes proposed in this book will cause only a *minimal* interruption of the present system.

To provide *free universal coverage for everyone in the country will not necessarily require imposing more taxes upon American citizens.* By making structural changes in the way we pay for our healthcare, we can provide free healthcare coverage for everyone in the country without raising taxes. This book provides one way of changing the system. The suggested modifications will not only lower the present healthcare spending, but will also correct the trend for future healthcare expenditures while improving the quality of care.

In lowering our healthcare prices, we will also lower the burden on businesses. Fundamental changes to our healthcare system are essential if we want to save our free-enterprise capitalistic economy by making it more competitive. Our businesses can lead the world again, if only we can reform healthcare. If we do not, the current situation threatens the survival of American business as well as our free enterprise system.

Although the main focus of the book is on the cost of healthcare, other problems with American healthcare are often overlooked by policymakers. One such problem is that the modern medicine has become very unsafe. Modern medicine treatments can be as risky if not riskier than the disease for which they are recommended.

Just as high cost is the result of a badly designed system, so is unsafe medicine a consequence of this same system. Closely related to the problem of risky medicine is the problem of medical malpractice. The prevalent view is that malpractice lawsuits are raising the prices of medicine. Overlooked is the fact that the lawsuits are a natural consequence of healthcare which has become riskier than the disease. Later in this book, we will examine the question of malpractice lawsuits to see if they are the cause higher prices or if this is just a myth.

In this book, the approach suggested for cutting malpractice lawsuits is to discourage unsafe medicine. This approach will automatically reduce lawsuits as well as the large number of fatalities that occur in our country because of medical mistakes.

Lastly, there is the problem of navigating the system. Insurance companies require that patients fill out forms even though the sick are in a feeble condition. Patients face the uncertainty of not knowing whether doctor-recommended treatments will be covered by their insurance. Too often, doctors make promises about their treatments while hiding the risks of these treatments. Often, insurance companies tell their patients the treatments are not worthy of coverage. Thus the sick find themselves between a rock and a hard place.

Under extreme circumstances, patients might have to choose between their life and a bill that could bankrupt them—even if the treatment saves their life. A good healthcare system should not require people to have to choose between their life and their lifetime possessions.

Healthcare reform provides a unique opportunity for sincere individuals from both political parties to come together and work on resolving this difficult issue. Those who are against altering the system based simply on the principle that it is a free-market system should take a second look at the problem. I anticipate that they will find this book useful. I hope we can change our healthcare system to bring down long-term costs and make it fair for everyone.

Even the die-hard fans of U.S. medicine and free markets find it hard to explain why a drug such as Lipitor manufactured by an American company should cost four times as much in the United States as in Canada.

CHAPTER 1

HEALTHCARE COSTS IN THE UNITED STATES COMPARED TO REST OF THE WORLD

How Americans Justify the High Cost of Their Healthcare

If you have used healthcare services in another country, you might already have some idea about the medical costs abroad. Since the United States has the highest healthcare costs in the world by far, no matter in which country your experience was with their healthcare services, you must have found the costs there much cheaper.

If you were in a European country such as Germany, France or England, you might have found the care as good or better than in the United States, but available at a fraction of the price. If you were in a Latin American or an Asian country, you must have noticed a very huge difference in healthcare prices.

This is not an uncommon experience.

When travelling abroad, Americans are often surprised by the low prices of healthcare in other countries.

Therefore, on their return home, it is natural for many to ask why the cost of medicine in America is so high although many other manufactured goods are cheaper and of better quality in the United States than they are in other developing countries.

Isn't healthcare based on the same system of free-markets that we use for the production of industrial goods? Yet why are the costs of same services and same drugs much higher in the United States than they are in other countries abroad?

Are other countries artificially controlling costs below fair prices through government intervention? Or, are we being defrauded by the healthcare industry?

These and similar questions about healthcare have managed to confuse many Americans.

For almost a century, America has been a world leader in manufacturing. We produce approximately 25 percent of the world's high quality industrial goods but at cheap prices. This is the result of the free-market capitalistic system that in general produces efficiency through fair competition.

Since we experienced phenomenal economic success by the adoption of the capitalistic system, we have adopted a similar system to provide healthcare services to the citizens of our country. But, in so doing, our healthcare prices have jumped to the highest levels in the world. According to ratings of several independent agencies such as the *Commonwealth Fund* and *The Organization for Economic Co-operation and Development* (*OECD*), our healthcare also ranks among the lowest in quality among all industrialized nations.

Whereas in other areas, the market economy is producing excellent results with high quality and low prices, in healthcare the prices have reached threateningly high levels. To make sense of the situation, most Americans have formed some opinions regarding the existing state of affairs. Although opinions vary regarding the overall quality of healthcare in the United States, most people have rationalized their beliefs to explain the high cost of medicine.

Below, are compared the medical costs in different countries. After comparisons, we will look at how Americans rationalize the high cost of medicine in their country. This will be followed by a discussion explaining why most of the popular views are incorrect.

By the end of this chapter you will probably begin to suspect that the high prices in United States are not due to the high quality of healthcare but possibly due to the faulty market structure of our system.

Here then is a comparison of costs in seven countries: United States, Canada, Germany, England, France, Argentina and Spain. All of the data presented in this chapter is taken from a report prepared by International Federation of Health Plans[7] and represents comparative international costs during the time covered by this report. The data is for illustrative purposes only.

Physicians' Fees in the United States Compared to Countries Around the World

Routine Office Visits

Table 1 shows that in the United States, a routine office visit to a doctor could cost you as much as $156.00. This cost is 4-10 times the cost for such a visit in Canada, Germany, or

Table 1

Cost of Routine Visits to Doctors' Offices in Various Countries

Routine Doctors Office Visit	
Country	Cost
US (Average)	$86.00
US (High)	$156.00
Canada	$39.00
Germany	$15.00
England	0.00
France	$31.00
Argentina	$8.00
Spain	$11.00

Table 2

Cost of Cataract Surgery in Various Countries

Cataract Surgery	
Country	Cost
US (Average)	$954.00
US (High)	$2,210.00
Canada	$502.00
Germany	$560.00
England	0.00
France	$1,158.00
Argentina	$120.00
Spain	$413.00

France. It is about 14-20 times what you would spend in Argentina or Spain. In Argentina, a visit to the doctor costs almost the same as a visit to McDonalds in the United States. In England, seeing your doctor is free because it is paid for by your taxes.

Even for more serious procedures the costs are more in the United States. Consider two such procedures: cataract surgery and hip replacement.

Table 2 shows a list of prices for cataract surgery in various countries. Although the price for this surgery in France is comparable to the average price in the United States the average price in the United States is almost double the price in Canada, Germany or Spain. It is eight times the cost in Argentina. In England, you do not pay anything.

Now consider hip replacement. Hip replacement costs are shown in Table 3. Here again, even though the average price for hip replacement in France is comparable to the price of hip replacement in the United States, it is more than three times the price in Canada or Germany. It is also almost three times of what it is in Spain and more than seven times the cost in Argentina. Once again in England it costs nothing. It is paid for by the taxes.

Prevailing Beliefs about Why Doctors' Services Cost so Much in America?

When Americans are asked why they think doctors' fees are higher in the United States, most people do not understand the reasons for this. However, if the question is reframed and they are asked why the doctors in the United States make so much

Table 3

Cost of Hip Replacement Surgery in Various Countries

Hip Replacement	
Country	**Cost**
US (Average)	$2,834.00
US (High)	$5,280.00
Canada	$815.00
Germany	$679.00
England	0.00
France	$2723.00
Argentina	$370.00
Spain	$1,071.00

more money than their counterparts in other professions or their counterparts in other countries, people do have opinions.

Most people believe, if doctors in America charge more than their counterparts in other countries or other professions then there must be a very good reason for it. Here are some of the common beliefs.

Common Belief No. 1: Doctors work long hours

Many people believe that doctors deserve to be paid more because they have to put in long hours. Often they have to be on call. Because of these requirements, people think that paying doctors well is justified.

But, there is a fundamental flaw with this commonly held belief. Any profession in which you are required to work long hours does not automatically entitle you to higher hourly wages for your work. For example, many laborers work long hours. Many maids and live-in helpers have to work long hours, but workers in these occupations make very little money. Even many other professionals such as physicists, politicians, and teachers also have to work long hours. Yet, their *average* incomes are much less compared to doctors.

Some nurses have to work longer hours than doctors and still do not make as much money as the doctors. Even in other countries doctors have to work equally long hours but that does not explain why their services in America cost more than their counterparts in other countries.

Common Belief No. 2: Medical education takes many years

Here is another common belief that is used to justify higher doctor income in the United States. Many Americans believe that since it takes several years to become a doctor, the higher income is justified.

But the flaw with this belief is that there are many other professions in which education can take a very long time. For example a Ph.D. in humanities on average can take about seven years or so after getting a Master's degree; yet, this type of education pays very little.

The length of education is not related to income of a profession, in the United States. As another example, a Ph.D. in engineering, physics or chemistry pays more than a similar degree in humanities though it takes less time to obtain. Therefore the length of education in itself cannot be the reason for the high incomes of doctors.

Common Belief No. 3: Doctors save lives.

Medicine is the type of profession where every now and then a doctor will have the opportunity to save a person's life. By the same token there will also be times when a doctor could make a mistake and cause a death. In fact in the practice of modern medicine many people die because of medical errors. Medical errors are the third leading cause of death in the United States.[8]

Even if you do believe that doctors deserve to be paid more because they save lives, so do doctors in other countries. Yet the doctors in other countries get paid much less. Canadian, German and British doctors all make much less. Doctors in many countries make only a fraction of what United States make but produce better results (1).

Even in our own country, there are other professionals who also save lives often by risking their own lives. These include firefighters, policemen and soldiers. Yet, their incomes are puny compared to that of doctors.

Common Belief No. 4: Doctors' work carries a lot of responsibility.

The way modern medicine is currently being practiced, it involves frequent surgeries and other risky procedures. In fact most medicine that is being practiced today carries with it a lot of risk. American doctors practice more high-risk medicine than the doctors in the other countries. In America, there are more surgeries and more high-tech procedures performed compared to other countries (Why this is so is a topic in itself and will be discussed later on in this book.)

Under current medical practices, it would be prudent to allow only people with a lot of training and education to be doctors.

But, once again, doctors in other countries carry just as much responsibility as their American counterparts. Yet the prices charged for the same procedures by the doctors in the United States are more than the prices charged by doctors in other countries as has been shown earlier in this chapter. So, this belief is also necessarily false.

Common Belief No. 5: American doctors are the best in the world.

Objective studies to evaluate which country has the best doctors in the world are almost non-existent. 'Best' is a very subjective belief. Most people come to that conclusion by assuming that since American doctors get paid more than in any other country therefore it must be because they are the best in the world. But this is like putting the cart before the horse. Just because locally sold and locally manufactured goods in the developing countries are very expensive for the native people, people in these countries do not assume that they are of better quality than those manufactured in America. Just because our doctors get paid more does not imply that they are the world's best.

Common Belief No. 6: American doctors get sued more so they must charge more to make up for the malpractice losses.

This argument is widely believed by many Americans. During his presidency, President George W Bush brought up this argument many times and portrayed it as the main cause of high prices of medicine in the United States.

Here is why this belief is also false: *Even after paying for the malpractice premiums, the doctors' incomes in the United States remain much higher than in other countries.* In other words the fees being charged by the doctors are high even after taking into account the malpractice premiums.

Chapters 2 and 4 will show why the doctors' services cost more in the United States. We will also see why limiting their liability will not make doctors lower their fees.

Malpractice damages were recently limited in Texas but the costs of medicine in Texas went *up, not down.* This is covered in more detail in Chapter 9.

What Else is Wrong with These Beliefs?

There is another very good reason why *any* of the above explanations cannot be true. All the above arguments assume that in United States a governing body overlooks the incomes of various professions and decides a ' fair ' income for each profession. If this were the case this government body would be saying "for all these reasons doctors *should* make more money."

In a free-enterprise system such as ours there is no government body (unlike in the former Soviet Union) that decides what is fair compensation for people in a particular profession. The vast majority of doctors in the United States are in private practice for themselves. *The income of doctors is being determined by the markets.*

If we want a true answer, then we will have to investigate the *peculiarities* of American healthcare markets that *allow* our doctors to charge higher fees compared to their counterparts in other parts of the world. This subject will be explored in detail in Chapters 2 and 4.

Hospital Costs around the World

It is not just the doctors' fees that are higher in the United States; it is also the hospital costs.

Table 4

The Cost of Hospital Stay in Various Countries

Hospital Stay	
Country	**Cost**
US (Average)	$14,427.00
US (High)	$45,902.00
Canada	$7.707.00
Germany	$4718.00
England	0.00
France	$4,715.00
Argentina	1,253.00
Spain	1,679.00

Table 5

The Cost of Hospital Stay per Day in Various Countries

Hospital Stay per Day	
Country	**Cost**
US (Average)	$3,612.00
US (High)	$14,306.00
Canada	$340.00
Germany	$554.00
England	0.00
France	$909.00
Argentina	$319.00
Spain	$470.00

The data in Table 4 shows that on average, it costs about twice as much for a hospital stay in the United States, as it costs in Canada and nearly three times of what it costs in Germany or France. It can be more than ten times the cost in Argentina. At the high end, a U.S. hospital stay can be about six times the stay in Canada and ten times the cost in France or Germany.

On a per-day basis, the cost differences between American hospitals and the rest of the world can be even greater. A look at Table 5 makes it clear. The table shows average costs of a per-day stay in a hospital in various countries.

In an average American hospital the daily cost can be more than ten times of that in Canada. It can be about four times of that in France and about six and a half times of the cost in Germany. In a more expensive hospital in the U.S. the cost could be fifteen times that of France and nearly twenty-six times that of Germany and an incredible forty-two times that of Canada.

Prevailing Beliefs About Why American Hospitals Cost More

Many people believe that the American hospitals are better equipped than the Canadian hospitals or the hospitals in other European countries such as France, Germany, or England or that we pay our nurses more, and therefore, the higher costs are perhaps justified.

In the end, it is the results that count and it is not the high-tech equipment or the income of doctors that is important for the patients. Despite the proliferation of high-tech equipment and despite the highest paid doctors in the world, American hospitals remain very dangerous places.[9]

The situation begs the question as to why is it that despite the best equipment and the most well-paid doctors in the world, American hospitals have the unsatisfactory safety record? This is a disturbing question, the answer to which will become clearer when we examine the general nature of healthcare markets in America.

Scans, Imaging Fees, and Drug Costs Around the World

Let us start with scans. Consider the abdominal scan.

As Table 6 shows, the average cost of a CT scan of the abdomen is $536 in the United States, but it could be as high as $1,564. It is $374 in Germany, the next most expensive. However, the cost in Canada is only $61, which is only one-twenty-fifth of the high cost in the United States. Table 6 gives the costs of abdominal CT scans in various countries in the world.

Similarly, referring to Table 7, the high cost of a head scan in the United States is $1,430. This is almost five times the next-highest cost of these scans in Germany, where on average they only cost $287. In Canada, the cost is only $65 per scan, which is less than 1/20th of that of the highest U.S. cost.

Prevailing Beliefs About Why Scans Cost More in the UnitedStates.

Even those who can justify high doctors' fees in America have trouble explaining high imaging and scanning prices. Why

Table 6
**Cost of a CT Scan of the Abdomen
in Various Countries**

Abdomen Scan	
Country	**Cost**
US (Average)	$536.00
US (High)	$1,564.00
Canada	$61.00
Germany	$374.00
England	$187.00
France	$179.00
Argentina	$85.00
Spain	$117.00

Table 7
Cost of a Head Scan in Various Countries

Head Scan	
Country	**Cost**
US (Average)	$464.00
US (High)	$1,430.00
Canada	$65.00
Germany	$287.00
England	$187.00
France	$179.00
Argentina	$60.00
Spain	$117.00

should the same scanning machine plugged in an American hospital or doctor's office command more payment

Most Americans don't have a good answer.

Drug Prices Around the World

As one last item of comparison, let us consider the cost of drugs in the United States. There are currently thousands of prescription and non-prescription drugs on the market. Of these we will consider the three top selling drugs in the world in the last few years. These are: Lipitor, Plavix and Nexium.

One of the most popular of these in the last few years has been Lipitor. It is a cholesterol-lowering drug manufactured by the American company Pfizer. Another best-selling drug that we will consider is Plavix. It is a blood-thinning drug used to inhibit blood clots in arteries. It is generally used to treat patients who have recently had a heart attack, stroke or arterial disease. It is manufactured by Bristol-Myers Squibb, a company headquartered in New York City. The last drug that we will consider is Nexium[10] which is used in the treatment of dyspepsia, peptic ulcer disease, and gastro-esophageal reflux disease. It is manufactured by the British company AstraZeneca, headquartered in London, United Kingdom.

Drug prices are an area where you will notice the most glaring differences in prices for identical products across the world. As Table 8 shows, even though the drug Lipitor[11] has been developed by an American company, its price in the United States is four times its price in Canada. Plavix, another drug manufactured by an American company costs ten times in the United States compared to what it costs in France, as Table 9

Table 8

Cost of Lipitor[12] in Various Countries

Lipitor	
Country	**Cost**
US Average)	$129.00
US (High)	$134.00
Canada	$31.00
Germany	$78.00
England	$39.00
France*	$0.43
Argentina	$38.00
Spain	$31.00

---

* The price of Lipitor in France is for the generic drug substitute Tahor

Table 9

Cost of Plavix in Various Countries

Plavix	
Country	**Cost**
US (Average)	$152.00
US (High)	$161.00
Canada	$76.00
Germany	$99.00
England	$57.00
France	$15.00
Argentina	$55.00
Spain	$80.00

Table 10

Prices of Nexium in Various Countries

Nexium	
Country	**Cost**
US (Average)	$186.00
US (High)	$339.00
Canada	$32.00
Germany	$136.00
England	$30.00
France	$3.00
Argentina	$21.00
Spain	$50.00

shows. Lastly, the drug Nexium in the United States costs more than sixty times its cost in France, as shown in Table 10.

Prevailing Views on the Prices of Drugs

Just as Americans are confused about the medical imaging costs, they are even more confused about the prices of drugs. Even the die-hard fans of U.S. medicine and free markets find it hard to explain why a drug such as Lipitor, manufactured by an American company costs four times as much in the United States as its cost in Canada.

Drug prices can invoke in U.S. consumers, a feeling of being cheated by the drug industry.

Conclusion

American healthcare prices are high across the board. Not only are the doctors' fees high, but the hospitals, scanning, imaging, and drugs – they all cost much more. Even after conjuring up reasons to justify higher payments for doctors and higher payments for our well-equipped hospitals, *most people cannot justify high imaging and drug prices.*

This leads us to believe that some flaws in our healthcare system are probably responsible for these high prices in *every* area of healthcare. This subject will be explored in the next chapter.

When people are not spending their own money to buy a product in a market, the market is not operating as a free-market.

CHAPTER 2

IS THE U.S. HEALTHCARE SYSTEM A FREE-MARKET?

"Insurance: An ingenious modern game of chance in which the player is permitted to enjoy the comfortable conviction that he is beating the man who keeps the table." – Ambrose Bierce.

The high U.S. healthcare costs pose a paradox: why does our free-market system, which logically should promote efficiency, produce higher prices, while in other countries with a lot of government regulation the prices are lower?

If we assume that free-markets* always produce efficiency, resulting in higher quality and lower prices, then two possible explanations come to mind. Either the governments in other countries are artificially lowering the prices of medicine and thus are being unfair to their healthcare providers, or the healthcare

---

*Throughout this book, the term "free-market" is being used in a very broad sense to mean a market that is capable of producing efficiency and fairness for both providers and consumers. This type of market is an efficient market in which the law of supply and demand holds.

providers in the United States are involved in some type of manipulation of the system.

Neither of these explanations is true, however. If we are willing to think more deeply, we will find that the answer to this predicament is quite simple. *When people are not spending their own money to buy a product in a market, the market is not operating as a free market.*

Even calling it a "market" is a bit of a stretch because the word "buying" implies people are using their own money in transactions. When we "buy" products by using the money from insurance companies, all the advantages of free markets vanish. Even the laws of economics (which are based on this implied assumption), melt down and fail.

This all-pervasive misunderstanding about a "free-market" lies behind most of our healthcare problems. This misunderstanding is responsible for problems that range from upward-spiraling healthcare costs including national budget problems, to the rising number of medically uninsured (though the numbers dropped after the passage of Obamacare), and a growing number of bankruptcies due to unpaid medical bills.

This misunderstanding is also the reason why, as a nation, we have spent years in debate and disagreement, but we have not been able to produce an acceptable solution to the problem. Healthcare reform has vexed American presidents since the days of President Harry S Truman.

A market in which all the players are private parties does not automatically make it a free-market. For example, a monopoly is not a free-market although the provider of goods in the market might be a private entity and the buyers might all be private individuals.

A free-market is an efficient market that is capable of producing wealth for providers as well as high-quality inexpensive products for the buyers. A free-market requires much more than that the players in the market are private entities. At the very least, it requires that buyers should spend *their own money*. This fact, so fundamental to the operation of free-markets, is assumed in the very definition of a market. To the authors of economic textbooks this fact is so obvious that they do not even feel the need to mention it in their texts.

In addition there are some other implicit and often unmentioned requirements that are necessary for free-markets to function properly. For example, another requirement for free-markets to work properly is that the consumers must be able to make sound decisions. This, in turn, requires that *consumers must be healthy enough to think clearly* in their own interest and *they should have an adequate knowledge about the value of the product they are buying.* However healthcare markets are very different from free-markets. A patient lying on the operating table in a semi-unconscious state is no position to bargain with his doctor to get the best price for his surgery.

In addition, in any market, a consumer must have a good knowledge of the product that he or she wants to consume. Once again in healthcare markets this is difficult to do. With the introduction of high technology into medicine, it is difficult for patients to keep up with medical knowledge.

Besides this, controversial information swirls around much in medicine. Therefore, most patients must rely on their doctors rather than decide for themselves.

Two Important Requirements for Free-Markets to Function Properly

Thus, the two conditions needed for free-markets to function that are not met in the American healthcare markets are the following:

1. Market participants must be healthy and knowledgeable enough to make intelligent decisions.

2. Market participants must use their own money when participating in markets.

Since the first requirement cannot be met in *any* healthcare market (sickness affects the decision-making capabilities of patients), this is a very good reason for not delivering healthcare through the market mechanisms. However, in America, a second mistake was also made to cover up the shortcoming posed by unhealthy market participants—this was the introduction of insurance to pay for their healthcare costs. The introduction of insurance in the healthcare arena solved one shortcoming of the system but has created another problem–unmanageable inflation.

The problem has become worse because we have chosen to pay doctors for the procedures that they decide to perform on patients without regards to the outcomes. We have also chosen to pay them more when the procedures are unsafe.

These payment practices have made medicine both *expensive* and *unsafe.*

The best way to illustrate these points is to take the example of a typical patient in our healthcare system who gets sick, and examine the various factors that encourage him and other market participants to behave in ways that affect both the price and the quality of care.

Consider what happens when a typical patient, who we will call 'John,' goes to the hospital. Even though the following situation represents only one such transaction in a market, the market is made up of numerous similar transactions from which the market acquires its character.

John Goes to the Hospital

A Typical Transaction in the Healthcare System

John is a forty-five-year-old hypothetical but typical patient in our American healthcare system. He is a middle-class citizen who works in a high technology company that provides his health insurance. He is married and has two children. Because of his stressful job and his obligations to his family, he does not have much time for exercise or to pay attention to his diet. His wife works, too, and neither of them have the time to cook every day.

The family combines some home cooking with a lot of fast food and other unhealthy meals eaten away from home. It is a typical American life. Everything seems to be going well for John until one day after coming home from work, shortly after eating his meal, he develops chest pains. His wife calls 911 and he is rushed to the hospital.

He is taken to the emergency room and treated. The doctor gives him the diagnosis. It was a mild heart attack and the drugs cleared the clot. But, it could happen again. He is given several options. John could choose to do nothing. Or he could choose to go for an angioplasty. A balloon (catheter) would be inserted into one of his arteries to open up the artery. Or, he could go for bypass surgery. The doctor recommends that he should take some action or he will be endangering his life.

As you will note, John has been given some choices. But, he is not healthy. He has been physically weakened by the experience. He has not been properly informed about the risks or benefits of the procedures. His capacity to decide is greatly diminished. His wife is not very knowledgeable about medicine either. Yet, his health is important to him and his family. He will have to decide quickly; essentially, he will be influenced by the recommendation of the doctors.

Finally, John decides to go for bypass surgery. He does not fully understand the risks or the benefits of his decision. Doctors have downplayed the risks of the procedure. An aspirin a day might have done him more good, but he goes for what his doctors recommend.

Therein is the biggest pitfall in our system. For all practical purposes, in critical situations and in life-threatening emergencies (or situations which we believe are life-threatening to us), we must rely on doctors' advice.

The doctors are paid on a fee-for-service basis, with *more payment for riskier procedures*. So, they have incentives to recommend riskier procedures. Whether they perform an expensive procedure or an inexpensive one, will not financially affect the patient very much because patients are only required to pay the co-pay. Most patients in such situations might opt for more expensive treatment thinking it might be better for them.

This type of collective behavior by the patients will raise the price of medicine in such a system while making healthcare unsafe. This also brings down the overall quality of medicine since *our system makes unsafe medicine more appealing to the doctors*. We will contrast this healthcare situation with another free-market choice, John buying a television set.

John Goes to Buy a Television Set

This is a typical transaction in a non-healthcare free market. There is no insurance company to help him out. He has an incentive to shop around because he has a limited income. Also, this time he is healthy and can think more clearly than when he was bedridden.

This is a very different situation than the one in which making a wrong decision could mean the difference between life and death. Although he might not understand how the television set functions, TVs come with a warranty. He also knows what features he wants in his TV. The various models of TV with all their features have been advertised in the brochures that he has perused.

Since all the manufacturers advertise their products, even before getting out of the home, he can compare the features, read reviews, talk to his friends and family, and become acquainted with the product. He is familiar with the companies that manufacture TVs. The companies have been in business for some time and have established a reputation for quality and customer satisfaction. They also offer service plans to reduce the risk of a bad investment. Nothing of the sort exists in the healthcare markets.

In short, he is much better equipped for the purchase of a television than he was when he was in the hospital and will pay only what is necessary. After all, it is his own money that he will be spending, not the insurance company's. The manufacturers must compete with each other in quality and price if they hope to sell their TV sets at all.

Healthcare Markets versus Free Markets:

Differences Between the two Situations

To gain an understanding of what drives our healthcare system, we will contrast these two situations.

1. Not spending one's own money

In first case, John is not spending his own money. For the most part, it is the insurance company that will pay. The co-pay to his insurance company is the same, no matter what the total cost is. He makes no effort to keep the costs down. In fact, he might want the best doctor or the most expensive treatment.

In the second case, he uses his own money. His funds are very limited and he must make sure that he gets the best value for his money.

2. *Not being healthy enough to make sound decisions*

In first case, he is not healthy enough to make decisions. Even if he had some knowledge of medicine, in his sorry state of health, he might not be able to decide what is best for him.

In the second case, when he goes to buy a TV, he has a clear mind and can make decisions about what type of a product he wants.

3. *Need*

In the first case, he is concerned with his health and there is a lot of risk. In the second case, the risk is much less–even if he makcs a wrong decision.

4. *Caregivers are not responsible for results*

In the first case, his caregivers are only responsible for using their best judgment as to the treatment he should have. They will be paid for the treatment they provide regardless of whether the treatment helps him or not. Since he is not spending his own money, *he does not care about the price of the treatment as long as there is a chance that it helps.*

In the second case, the manufacturers of the television sets offer some type of a warranty.

As is clear, our current system is a very inefficient way to control costs because the consumer is not concerned about the price, does not understand what he is buying, and is not healthy enough to make sound decisions. To make things worse, the provider is being paid not for the results but what procedures he or she performs. His doctor will get paid even if John dies due to complications of the surgery.

Two Pillars of our Healthcare Payment System and the Resulting Consequences

The following two items are features of our payment system: like its two pillars.

1. Doctors are paid on a fee-for-service basis regardless of health benefits. They make more money if treatments are unsafe.

2. Payments to providers are made by third-party private health insurance.

Like pillars that support a building, these two principles form the basis for the functioning of our healthcare markets and are responsible for various problems in our system.

The healthcare system that covers most Americans, whether under or over the age of 65 uses these pillars.[13] The only difference is that the Americans over the age of 65 are covered by government insurance under Medicare rather than through private insurance. The system was not designed by policymakers using a comprehensive well planned policy. It is an outcome of historical needs that were fulfilled by private providers at various times in our national past. The reason we continue to use private providers and payers for healthcare, is that as a nation we believe that private enterprise is the best way of providing for all the needs of our society.

It is the private ownership of businesses that made America prosperous. Therefore, we have chosen to continue using private providers also for the delivery of healthcare.

But the fee-for-service feature of our system turns doctors into business people who are tempted to perform more of the unsafe procedures to make more money. When this payment method is used in combination with private insurance–where people are not concerned with the cost–it is a recipe for uncontrollable costs and overuse of unsafe medicine.[14]

Another possible way of paying doctors is to pay them for the health-benefit they provide. Such a system would be fairer to the patients, but difficult to implement.

Under such a system, far less effort (such as dietary advice) by the doctor could end up being more beneficial to the patient than a surgery (a much more difficult procedure). Such a fee-for-health system would have correct incentives, although patients and their insurance companies might feel uncomfortable paying out large sums for doctors' verbal advice but paying less for complex surgeries. Another problem is that it is difficult to measure health. So, under such a system, some questions will be hard to answer: did the patient get better by

healing powers within his or her body or by doctor's advice?
Did the patient cooperate with the doctor in the
treatment plan or ignore the doctor's recommendations?

Therefore such a system has never been suggested. The current
system continues to be practiced with its inflationary
consequences. Therefore, it is worthwhile to get some estimate
of how much inflation the current system is causing and what
type of pattern of inflation results because of it.

How Much Healthcare Inflation Is Created by Perverse Doctor Incentives and Insurance ?

Health Insurance as an Addition to the Nation's Money Supply

It is best to view the healthcare insurance as an increase in the
nation's money supply. Every time consumers buy a health
insurance policy, they effectively create an estate for
themselves. In other words, if the policy has a lifetime limit of
say a million dollars, it is like owning a million dollars in
reserve that can be used to pay medical expenses if they get
sick.

All a person has to do to hold on to his million dollar estate is to
pay the monthly premiums to the insurance company.

Just as the banks can expand nation's money supply by giving
out lines of credit, buying health insurance can do the same. In
this respect, insurance is no different from a line of credit
issued by a bank. A line of credit to a business often comes
with the understanding that the money will be used for
business-related expenses. Similarly the money from health

insurance can be used only by a licensed healthcare physician in case the insured is sick.

Since the insurance money can be spent only on healthcare expenses, it results in inflation *only* in the healthcare markets. This is why the *healthcare costs are going up faster* than the rate of general inflation.

Unlike business owners who must be careful about spending their lines of credit because eventually they would have to pay back the loan, patients have no such worry. Whereas insurance should ideally be used for critical healthcare needs, patients believe they can improve their health by going to a doctor. Doctors are only too happy to oblige. Thus, both patients and doctors have an incentive to use up the insurance dollars, causing excessive spending.

Whether someone is healthy or sick is sometimes a judgment call made by patients or their doctors. No one's health can possibly be perfect, according to the high standards set by the healthcare industry.[15] Such high standards provide doctors an opportunity to provide some treatment to just about anyone.

Any licensed healthcare provider who can promise better health can tap into this vast money pool and get a piece of it for himself or herself. The highly specialized and technical nature of medicine makes it easy to sell expensive healthcare to patients whether or not it is needed.

This expanded money supply available for medical needs has caused a spiral of inflation for healthcare services. Over the past several years, the rate of inflation in medicine has been two to three times the rate of general inflation.

One can easily observe the perverse effects of the system on distorted prices in healthcare markets. In today's market where the median yearly household income in the United States is approximately $53,657, people sometimes get heart surgeries that can run up to $500,000 or more in cities such as New York.[16] If we did not have a system where payments are made by insurance companies, such high prices would not be sustainable, so the inflation we are experiencing would not ensue.[17] This shows how payment systems can impact what medical procedures are performed and at what costs.

In case of open-heart surgeries, it has not even been demonstrated that they are more effective than other treatment regimes. Yet, these are performed frequently in the United States. They are a prime example of wasteful, expensive, and unsafe medicine.

If patients were required to pay for healthcare expenditures from their own savings, it would be impossible for these surgeries to cost that much. It is doubtful if the doctors would recommend them or even if these types of surgeries would ever have been developed.

The newly passed Affordable Care Act of 2010 does not allow the insurance companies to put lifetime limits on insurance benefits. Thus, it allocates virtually unlimited amounts of money into the healthcare system. *This provision in the Affordable Care Act has the potential to raise future healthcare costs.* Even though the new law relieves the burden on the sick by ensuring that they will be covered no matter what the lifetime cost of their disease, it also creates an opportunity for unethical healthcare providers to make virtually unlimited amounts of money and cause an upward spiral in prices.

In Chapter 6, we will discuss a better way to deliver medicine not hampered by predicaments such as these.

Hockey-Stick Healthcare Inflation Curve

As we have seen, the incentives present in our system have resulted in accelerating inflation in healthcare costs for the last several decades. The pattern of this inflation is beautifully captured in the 'hockey stick curve' plotted in Figure 2.1 using the data provided by The Centers for Medicare and Medicaid Services for years 1960 to 2012 (2).

Figure 2.1 shows that not only are healthcare costs increasing every year, but their rate of increase also keeps on increasing.[18]

Any changes that we make to our healthcare policy must focus on altering the shape of this curve so it can trend downward. If we change our healthcare policy in ways that do not alter the shape of this curve, our efforts will be of no avail in controlling future costs.

As we will discuss in Chapter 5, many of the popular proposals put forward by legislators for reforming our healthcare system ignore this important point. Though some proposals will bring down the costs *in the year these are implemented*, they do nothing to eliminate the fundamental reasons for the hockey-stick shape of this cost-curve.

The Hockey-Stick Curve

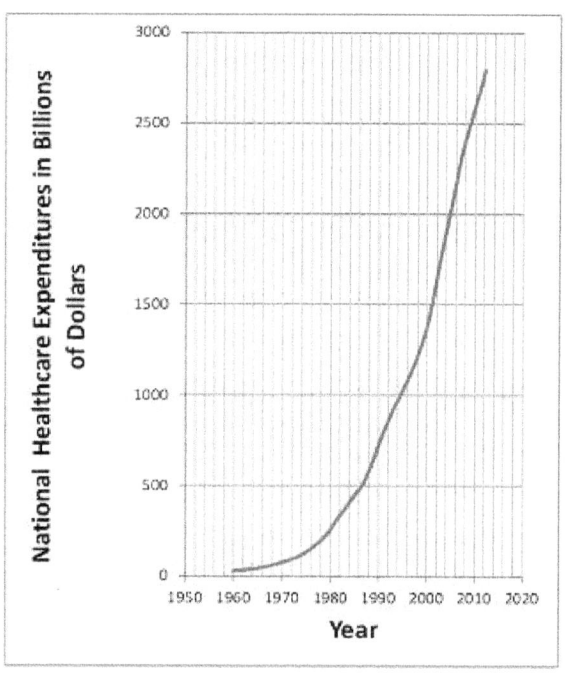

Figure 2.1 National Healthcare Expenditures 1960-2012

Why do Healthcare Costs Have a Hockey-Stick Shape?

It is critical to understand what is making the rate of healthcare costs increase each year, and why the rise in costs has the shape shown in Figure 2.1? Therefore, in the paragraph below I would like to speculate on the reasons for the shape of this curve.

Our system causes demands for medical services to increase as their cost increases. If a medical procedure is more expensive, patients want it more, because the insurance will pay[19] for it. Patients incorrectly believe that more expensive procedures must be better for them. Doctors do not like to discourage patients' demands because they stand to gain from them. They do not faithfully inform patients of the risks of medicine. It is this *increased demand for more expensive healthcare* (while being shielded from its cost) that causes this hockey-stick shaped curve. This phenomenon is opposite to what happens in free markets where *demand decreases* with *higher* prices.

When in Chapter 5 we examine the various proposals for healthcare reform, it will be important to pay attention to this curve. Any lasting solution for lowering costs *must* take into account the underlying factors shaping this curve.

The next chapter will examine the incentives of various players in the healthcare market and show how these incentives have a synergetic effect to produce high costs in addition to introducing some other peculiarities into our system.

Thou shalt not be allowed to heal unless thou put a patented and potentially harmful substance in your mouth that maketh a profit for someone else

CHAPTER 3

HOW INCENTIVES TO VARIOUS MEDICAL PROVIDERS AFFECT THE PRICES AND THE TYPE OF MEDICINE THAT IS PRACTICED

The previous chapter considered the role of incentives on doctors in the healthcare system. But, there are also other players in the market such as hospitals, drug companies, medical device manufacturers, and insurance companies. Their incentives also play a role in shaping the markets.

We pay private medical providers in ways similar to those we use to pay doctors. Providers get paid for *each* service they render or *each* product they sell. Though this method of paying seems perfectly logical, it has its down side in the healthcare markets. It incentivizes private providers to sell *more* of their products and services in order to make higher profits.

In the non-healthcare markets, this urge to sell can be a positive force that can drive the economic engine of a country. It works exceptionally well for producing wealth in any country where such a system is implemented. However, in healthcare markets, this system has the effect of overwhelming the citizens with *too much* unnecessary medicine.

Selling medical services and drugs with harmful side effects to unhealthy consumers (patients),[20] who do not completely understand what they are getting and whose bills will be paid by insurance, is a recipe for unnecessary medicine as well as spiraling costs.

At first it might appear that drug companies, hospitals, and medical device manufacturers–all have incentives to pressure doctors to sell more of their products or services. But the truth is a bit more complex. The doctors' incentives and the incentives of other providers are aligned so that all can help each other in making more money. In a system that relies on insurance to pay the providers, even the patients want more medicine. So, incentives of all these players have a synergetic effect that inflates the costs.

The only other players in the market, who have an incentive in lowering the costs, are the insurance companies, that pay the medical providers. Insurance companies, therefore, stand alone on the other side of the fence and are in a position to check the costs. But, as we shall see, because of their unique role as payers, they are also much despised by all the other players in the market.

The following discussion focuses on doctors, drug companies, hospitals, and private insurance companies. Because incentives of manufacturers of medical devices are similar to those of drug companies, they are not discussed separately.

Doctors' Incentives

Doctors' incentives play the most important role in our system, because doctors are at the forefront of the system. It is their responsibility to decide how much and what kind of medicine to dispense. Drug companies cannot sell many of their drugs unless the doctors write prescriptions. Even hospitals cannot sell their services unless doctors admit patients. Because doctors control the sales of goods and services of other providers, they bear the primary responsibility for the amount of medicine that is consumed nationally.

Therefore doctors have an enormous influence on the total national expenditures on healthcare. Since they are in the driver's seat, any effort to reform the system must pay special attention to reforming the incentives for doctors.

Let us see how doctors' incentives interact with the incentives of other providers to create a dynamic that affects healthcare costs as well as the *type* of medicine that is being practiced.

Under our current system, doctors enjoy a *mutually profitable* relationship with drug companies *as well* as with hospitals. Just as the drug companies and hospitals are dependent upon doctors for their income, the *doctors, too, in turn, are dependent upon these industries* for their income.

It is in doctors' financial interest to work in cooperation with the pharmaceutical companies as well as the hospitals. Any sale made by any drug company or any use of hospital facilities involves a payment to the doctor, too, since the doctor must first write a prescription or be engaged in the use of the hospital facilities.

Let us first consider doctors' relationship to drug companies. Drug companies depend upon the doctors to sell their drugs because most drugs cannot be sold unless a doctor writes a prescription. However, the dependence of doctors on drug companies might be less obvious to the reader. Therefore, this point needs elaboration, and is discussed in more detail in the next section.

In this section it will suffice to say that doctors prefer to use drugs rather than *safer* natural substances because by using drugs, they can exercise greater control over their patients.[21] Since many drugs have serious side effects, a doctor is required to write prescriptions and to monitor the patient for safety.

Just as doctors need the drug companies for them to make money, doctors also need hospitals. The current medical system has *evolved* to require expensive high-technology machines, which have become a necessary part of the medical practice.

Doctors need imaging machines such as MRI machines, X-ray machines, and CAT scan equipment for diagnosis. They also need operating theaters in which they can perform surgeries and nursing staff to take care of their patients and watch them for possible problems after a surgery. Therefore, in order for surgeons to make money, they need hospitals filled with equipment and staff.

Similarly, hospitals need doctors. They cannot rent their facilities unless the doctors are willing to admit their patients to them.

Why Are Drugs Used in Modern Medicine?

Another consequence of doctor incentives

One of the most misunderstood areas of our healthcare system is the role that the drugs play in modern medicine. Most people view drugs as an indispensable part of modern medicine. Very few people realize that prescription drugs are the *result of incentives that are inherent in the fee-for-service system for payment to doctors.*

In a fee-for-service system, to make money all doctors need to sell their services. This also means that doctors can make more money from their patients if they exercise *control* over them. This means using only those treatments that require a licensed professional. One way to do this is to prescribe drugs rather than using non-prescription alternatives. The patient must return to the doctor to get a prescription refilled, and the doctor must monitor the patient for any possible harmful effects of medication since all drugs carry potentially harmful side effects (that is why they are sold through prescriptions).

Besides allowing doctors to exercise control over their patients, drugs also help a doctor in alleviating the necessity of completely understanding a patient's illness. Rather than spending time with the patients to get to the root of their problems, the doctor will simply write a prescription to alleviate the symptoms the patient is having. For example, even when doctors do not understand the cause of their patients' pains, they often prescribe painkillers. If they cannot put out the fire, they can, at least, turn off the fire alarm. Writing a prescription is also a way to end a visit quickly and tangibly—patients walk out with something in their hands.

The drugs also allow doctors to see more patients in a short time. Using drugs, doctors can treat the patient quickly (if only at a symptomatic level) giving the impression to the patient that the patient is being healed. The payments doctors receive from the insurance company are based on how many patients a doctor sees rather than how much time the doctor spends with each patient. The more patients a doctor can see the more money the doctor can earn.

In addition, in a third party payment system, doctors have to make sure that their treatments (procedures, tests, and drugs) align with the requirements of the insurance companies and are recognized as valid medical treatments. Otherwise, the insurance company can refuse to pay for the patient's visit.

If a doctor suggests garlic or turmeric for healing, it might raise eyebrows at the insurance company. Even spending the time necessary with the patient to pin down underlying causes that might be causing patients ailments might not carry any extra payment for the doctor.

An insurance company claims adjustor sitting in another city cannot observe what is going on in a doctor's office. All the health insurance company recognizes is a *properly filled out claim form.* A disease must be named on the form and properly coded, and standard drugs for that disease must be prescribed.

Thus, in a system where payments are paid by a third party, Safer natural products such as herbs are not a *recognized billable item,* though the prescription drugs are.

Effect of Widespread Doctors' Practices on Patient Expectations

Because of the near-universal use of drugs by doctors, even patients have come to expect them as a matter of course. Remember the last time you visited your doctor? Chances are that you walked out of the doctor's office with either your doctor ordering some tests for you, performing a procedure, or writing a prescription. Or perhaps all three.

All these services have certain things in common. These are the services that can only be performed by licensed practitioners. These are also the services for which an insurance company will pay.

For these reasons, some or all of above services are performed nearly every time a patient goes to see a doctor. Because of their widespread use, patients have come to expect them, too. If you went to a doctor who did none of these things but simply discussed your condition and then sent you home simply by advising you on diet and exercise, or suggested some herbs and spices that you could buy without a prescription, you might feel you did not get your money's worth.

The advice that this doctor gave you might have been the best piece of advice for you. It might have required sacrifice on the part of your doctor because it is very unlikely that he or she would receive any payment from the insurance company for *only* giving advice.

Still, it is possible that it might not have satisfied you. Any deviation from this practice can seem unsatisfactory to the patient. Thus, the practice of doctors writing prescriptions has become an established practice; not only does it help doctors but also satisfies patients' expectations.

Such widespread practice has convinced our society that drugs are necessary for any form of healing.

Effect of Laws Requiring Prescriptions

But how did such widespread use of prescription drugs get started? In the United States, a key event that encouraged greater use of drugs was the passage of Durham-Humphrey Amendment in 1951.[22] It required doctor's prescriptions for the sale of certain drugs. Prior to the passage of this law, prescriptions were not required for the purchase of medicinal drugs.

This law empowered doctors but limited the freedom of patients and as we have seen, it offered doctors a way to control patients and earn greater income. This provided further incentives for doctors to use mostly drugs in their practice rather than safer substances. Perverse incentives made doctors turn their backs to the foremost advice of the father of medicine Hippocrates who said "first do no harm."

Because the fee-for-service system for payment to doctors (as well as requirements that many drugs be bought by prescription only) is used not only in America but to a lesser or greater degree in many other countries in the world, the same incentives as in our system have also guided the behavior of healthcare providers in other countries. Thus, drugs are considered a necessity not only in the United States but all over the developed world.

The effect has been so profound that prescription drugs are now considered an integral part of modern medicine. It is unfortunate that *the use of safer of substances is now perceived as being quackery.* I am sure if Hippocrates were alive today and was practicing safe medicine, even he would be labeled as a quack by the same medical profession that he helped establish. What is really sad is that there are some people in our society who have even begun to believe that unless drugs have serious side effects, they won't be effective.[23]

My Experiences with Alternative and Herbal Medicine

Erosion of my Trust in Modern Medicine

Like most people, for years I had believed that the reason natural herbs or safer treatments were not used by doctors is that they were ineffective. I had always told myself that our doctors are well educated and well versed in the established body of medical science and have spent years of training in their field, so they must be in a position to know the best methods of healing.

However, a few positive experiences with herbal medicine in the last few years have changed my mind. These experiences have been one of the major factors that have altered my perception of modern medicine and were also a factor that prompted the writing of this book.

My first experience in alternative medicine concerns my wife. My wife has had lifelong allergies, which after an episode of unrelated illness became much worse. For several weeks she suffered from nonstop coughing, sneezing, and a runny nose. The situation became unbearable for both of us. She had already been taking allergy medication for about twenty years, so trying out more medication was not an option.

I asked her if she were willing to try something entirely different. I had heard that sometimes milk avoidance can relieve allergies. She abstained from drinking milk for a few days. The results were dramatic. Her years of allergies all disappeared in *three* days. In the three years since she stopped drinking milk, her allergies have not returned.

Another experience that helped me take a positive view of alternative medicine also concerns my wife. Some time ago she came down with case of shingles. Shingles is a viral disease caused by the virus Herpes Zoster. Doctors told me that antiviral drugs are not effective unless they are taken immediately after the attack. Since some days had already passed after the attack, the drug option was not available. Since she was in intense pain, I gave her a few drops of Olive Leaf Extract (OLE). An acquaintance of mine had told me that Olive Leaf Extract can be effective for herpes as well shingles. After taking a few drops every day, she started to recover.

Her improvement was particularly surprising to me since many doctors had told me that not many drugs are useful against viruses. In general, the medical profession has created an impression that most viral infections are untreatable just because there are not many anti-viral *drugs*. However *there is only half-truth in these assertions.*

Even though there are not very many anti-viral *medications* on the market, there are many anti-viral *substances* in nature. Studies have shown that garlic, olive leaf, turmeric, and numerous other natural substances have anti-viral properties

(3). Use of these substances can be extremely effective for viral infections. For those readers who are interested in reading more about herbal medicine, see the references at the end of this book, especially (3) and (4). A comprehensive free source of research papers on the use of natural substances as well as other medical literature can also be found at http://www.ncbi.nlm.nih.gov/pubmed.

In my own experiments with herbs, I have found them extremely effective. I used to become sick two-to-three times every year during the flu season. But, in the last ten years, I have added uncooked garlic, turmeric, olive leaf extract, and thyme to my diet and have not experienced any flu or cold ever since.

These experiences have thoroughly convinced me that there are many safer cheaper and easily available cures that are being ignored by doctors because of the perverse incentive system. Use of these herbal and safer substances does not require a doctor's prescription or supervision. These treatments do not give the doctor control over the patient. Therefore, they are not used nor encouraged by doctors.

If we want to bring down healthcare costs, we must change incentives in a way that changes the *type of medicine* that is being practiced. This fact will be especially relevant when we consider solutions for improving our healthcare system. More discussion on this topic is included in Chapter 8.

Drug Company Incentives

The need of doctors to have prescription drugs at their disposal has created a large (and powerful) drug industry. The pervasive use of drugs by doctors for every imaginable ailment has advanced the interests of this industry.

The main method used in the United States for encouraging the research and development of drugs is to award patents for the development of drugs. Most developed countries of the world also have the same policy to encourage the development of new drugs. However, when the patent system is used to encourage the development of drugs, it has an impact on overall healthcare costs unlike when patents are used to encourage innovation of other consumer goods.

Because of the unique nature of drugs, the drug companies must use sales techniques that are more subtle than those used by manufacturers of other consumer goods. The system has not only resulted in high prices, but the sales techniques employed have had an effect on medical education as well as on society's beliefs about health, sickness, and disease prevention.

The Patent System's Effect on Drug Costs

First, consider how the system of granting patents to drug companies to encourage research in drug development is affecting drug prices. The patent system for the encouragement of the development of drugs is a policy choice. The philosophy behind the granting of patents is that it provides financial incentives to private researchers to develop drugs without cost to taxpayers. Thus, it is considered cheaper to develop drugs in this way than for the government to get involved in drug research. But, this view is too simplistic and ignores several facts.

Although the potential for making profits motivates researchers to work hard to develop drugs, it does have some disadvantages and is not the only way to encourage research. The granting of patents requires little or no public money during the drug development phase but gives the researchers a limited-time monopoly over the sale of their product. They can thus charge exorbitant prices for these drugs because drugs are perceived to be lifesaving, and their cost is paid through the deep pockets of insurance companies.

The short patent-expiration periods further contribute to higher prices. Drug patents expire within twenty years from the date they are filed. The government has deliberately kept the patent periods short so that the drugs can come into the public domain quickly and be made available to everybody at a *low* cost. However, the system also has had some unintended consequences that tend to drive *up* the costs further. These short patent-expiration periods put an additional pressure on drug companies to recoup their costs and make as much additional profit as possible *within* this allotted time period. The drug companies raise the prices to unreasonably high levels during this period. Selling drugs at these prices often does not pose a problem, since drugs are perceived to be lifesaving, are sheltered from competition, and the cost is borne by the insurance companies.

Consider the following examples. The cancer drug Gleevec (manufactured by Novartis), which is used for chronic myeloid leukemia, entered the market in 2001 at a price of about $30,000/ year. At the time of this writing, its cost has increased about three times since its introduction (5). Similarly, the cancer drug Avastin can cost between $42,800 to $55,000 for a typical patient (6), (7), but the benefit of the drug has been judged to be minimal. A study published in the *New England Journal of Medicine* showed that Bevacizumab (the generic name for Avastin) extended life by only 4.7 months.

Drug companies can afford to charge such high prices (for drugs that show little benefit) that more than compensate the companies for their research only because we have a system that uses insurance dollars to pay for the drugs.

If Americans were required to pay for these drugs using their own money not many people would be able to afford them. No drug company would dare to quote such high prices. No such drugs would be developed. Medicine would be cheaper and probably more effective because people would not be able or willing to spend money for questionable benefits.

Under a different system, the types of drugs people would be taking and prices of these drugs would be very different. This is a good example of how the payment and incentive system shapes the nature of the medicine being practiced. Thus, the intellectual property rights and the patent system that works well in many other areas of the economy, such as for producing innovative products in consumer goods, does not work too well when it comes to drugs.

Not only does the system make drugs very expensive, but because the government pays for almost 40 percent of the total national dollars spent on healthcare[24] (through Medicaid, Medicare, the VA, and other government programs), it must buy and thus pay for the these drugs at hugely inflated prices. Any of the taxpayer money that was supposedly saved by assigning the research to private drug companies must be paid back to drug companies with huge profits on top of everything else.

All this not only adds to the government costs (*and thus to the taxpayer costs*) but also adds to the costs of those who pay for their healthcare through private insurance. The people paying for drugs through private insurance end up paying *twice*. First, in terms of higher taxes that now must be paid to support the higher government costs for programs such as Medicare, Medicaid and the VA. Second, their premiums to private insurance companies are also higher because of the higher drugs prices.

If the high cost of the patent system were the only drawback of the system, it might still be tolerable. However, a bigger shortcoming of the system is that the patent system encourages research into only those substances *that are patentable*. In nature, an abundance of substances, such as herbs, spices, foods, and vitamins, have healing properties and often are much safer and cheaper to use. But, under the patent system of developing drugs coupled with the doctors' incentives for using prescription medicines, we are ignoring these vital cheaper and safer alternatives. There is strong evidence that effective and safer therapies do exist even for serious diseases such as cancer. For more information, see books such as (8), (9), (10), (11), and a growing list of other excellent books.

Problems also arise from drug companies' needs to market their somewhat unique consumer product. They must market their product in a way that hides their profit motives from the public and impress upon society that their patented products are offered *solely* for the public good. They have thus played a role in creating the impression that the drugs are the *only* substances that can heal. *In addition, they must also use very innovative ways to create demand.*

In Chapter 4, we will see what *types of sales techniques* these companies use to accomplish these goals and how their sales and marketing techniques are having an adverse effect on medical education, as well as on our understanding of health, disease, and prevention.

Then, in Chapter 6, we will discuss how we can change the entire system of delivering healthcare by changing the incentives of various players in the system. Healthcare reform must involve reform of the drug industry, too. This includes re-evaluating the policy of issuing patents and requiring prescriptions for drug sales. We also must examine alternative methods of encouraging research other than solely through the granting of patents. We must also examine whether we must continue requiring *prescriptions* for the purchase of medications.[25] We must also examine whether we have alternatives to the fee-for-service payments for doctors.

Hospital Incentives

History of the Payment System to Hospitals

The high prices charged by American hospitals are not only the result of present day incentives but are also the result of mistakes made by insurers in the past. Due to their lack of understanding, insurers *inadvertently* managed to *encourage* hospitals to charge higher prices.

To understand why the hospital costs in America are so high is to get a mini lesson in healthcare economics. A badly instituted system of the past with perverse incentives managed to accelerate the costs, resulting in the high prices of today. Here is how it happened:

In the early days (in 1950s) when private health insurance was evolving as a means of payment for healthcare,[26] third-party payers had a conviction that even though hospitals were privately owned, they should not exist solely to make profits. Insurers believed that hospitals were supposed to be rendering a service to the society and should not be run like other profit-motivated businesses. Insurance companies, therefore, decided to pay hospitals for their costs plus a small profit based on the percentage of their costs. This proved to be a bad idea based on wishful thinking of the insurance companies. Just because the payers believed that hospitals should not exist solely to make money did not mean that the hospitals shared in that belief.

The only way for hospitals to make more profits was to increase their expenses. Hospitals could make high guaranteed profits without any risk as long as they were willing to spend indiscriminately. Thus began a race among hospitals to acquire new equipment, more staff, and better facilities. It did not matter how much money they spent, it would now be paid for by the insurers.

On top of their expenditures, hospitals would get a neat profit as a percentage of the money they spent. They faced no risk. The more they spent, the more profits they made. The race to spend was on. The only impediment was to think of new ways to spend.

During this period, hospitals were transformed from bare bones facilities to places with more luxurious accommodations with many amenities: comfortable beds and televisions in rooms resembling motel rooms. Not surprisingly, hospital costs rose during this period at an alarming rate. For example, in 1970s, federal spending on Medicare Part A rose *five fold* from $5 billion to $25 billion.

Then, the third party payers realized their mistake. It was time to do something about the problem. The Health Care Financing Administration (HCFA)*, the government agency responsible for paying for Medicare, changed the payment system. Instead of paying the hospitals on basis of expenses, it decided to pay them on a system based on Diagnostic Related Groups (DRGs). In other words, the hospitals would be paid according to the sickness that was diagnosed for the patient.

Under the new system, it would not matter how many days the patient stayed in the hospital or what the hospital expenses were. The hospital would be paid a flat sum based on the diagnosis.

While this method of payment has proved better than the previous one, and was effective in slowing down the costs, it came too late. The change came at a time when the hospital costs had already risen to high levels, and this new system of payment still suffers from many shortcomings discussed in the following paragraphs.

Currently, hospital expenses in the United States are several times the expenses of those in other countries as we noted in Chapter 1. At the time of this writing, a ten-day stay in a Northern Virginia hospital can cost you $250,000 or more.

*Now known as Centers for Medicare and Medicaid Services (CMS)

Even though the present system of payment based on DRG groups is better than the previous system based on expenses, it none-the-less suffers from the same flaws that every private for-profit system must suffer from. Since hospitals are private entities, they are driven by the money motive. When the system of payment was changed to a DRG payment system, the hospitals responded by cutting the number of days patients were kept in the hospitals. If you have recently been in a hospital and were discharged sooner than you you should have, now you know the reason.

As long as the motive for a service is money, the behavior of the caregivers will not be geared toward the need of the patient but toward earning more money. The method of payment determines the behavior. If the payment is based on how many services are provided, then the tendency of the hospital would be to sell you more of these. On the other hand, if we pay a flat payment then the hospitals would maximize their profits by providing the least possible service for the flat payment.

Finally, let us consider another player in the market: the private insurance companies.

Private versus Government Insurance:

What Works Better for Healthcare?

No matter what system we use for providing healthcare to our citizens (whether we continue to use the present fee-for-service system or change to another system), one thing is certain: we would need a third party to pay for those who are sick. By its very nature, sickness creates a financial need but takes away the ability to earn. Sickness also takes away patients' ability to effectively participate in the free markets.

We cannot change these fundamental facts about sickness although we *can* do something about how we choose the third-party payer and the method we use to base our payments to doctors and to healthcare providers. The third party can be a private insurance company or it can be government. The payments can be based on fee-for-service basis or some other basis such as a flat fee.

The question that needs to be examined is that even if we do not change anything else in our system except that we make the government the sole insurer[27] instead of private insurance companies, can this result in a reduction in our total healthcare costs?

The United States is unique among the countries in the world in that most people under the sixty-five years of age pay healthcare providers through private insurers. In most other countries, the payer is the government (for most of the population). Could it be that the private insurance system in the United States is inadvertently raising healthcare costs? That is, even if we continued to pay our doctors on a fee-for-service basis, but simply mandated that the government would be the sole insurer, could it result in lower costs?

To comprehend this issue, we need to understand the insurance business. Insurance is different from most other businesses. Whereas most businesses become more efficient because of privatization, the benefits of privatization to the insurance industry are minimal, because the insurance industry performs many functions similar to those performed by governments in capitalistic economies.

Insurance companies collect money from mixed pools of healthy and sick and give it to those who are sick. This is the main function of an insurance company. It is very similar to what governments do. Governments collect taxes from the rich and middle class and give the money collected back to help the poor or spend it on society's common needs.

Private insurance companies have some disadvantages compared to the government if government acted as an insurer. First, because private companies need to make a profit, they must charge higher premiums. Second, if government is the only insurer, then the government enjoys a monopoly position as a payer; therefore, it has more control over how much it wants to pay the medical providers. On the other hand, private insurance companies do not have that luxury. They must compete with each other as payers.

If an insurance company does not pay its doctors well, the doctors can refuse to accept payments from this insurance company. The company then will be less popular with those who want to buy insurance. *Therefore, by necessity, private insurance companies must pay more to the healthcare providers.*

In the single-payer system in Canada, the government is the sole insurer, and because of its monopoly powers as a payer, *it can better control the fees for certain services to doctors.*[28] (Canadian governments can and do bargain with their doctors over what they will pay for doctors' services.) This is one of the reasons Canadian healthcare costs are lower than those in the United States.[29]

In addition, private companies, in general, are less trusted when it comes to insurance. Remember that when it comes to putting our money in savings accounts in banks, we trust the banks only because the Federal Deposit Insurance Corporation (FDIC)[30] is backed by the U.S. government. We trust government because, in the ultimate analyses, government is us.

When it comes to health insurance, private insurance companies are also more likely to deny payments for certain treatments to patients to maximize their profits. If government denies coverage, it would not likely be for profit but for more genuine reasons such as ineffective treatments.

The public option was discussed as a part of the Affordable Care Act, but it did not pass because private insurers feared it would become overwhelmingly popular and put them out of business. This brought home the point that people trust government more than the private sector on important issues such as healthcare.

Had the public option passed and had it become popular, out-competing private insurance companies, it could have turned our system into one similar to the Canadian system. This might have resulted in a slightly better system than what we have now, but it would not have solved all our problems. Most hospitals in America are private, independent and very expensive. In Canada the hospitals (even the private hospitals) are strictly controlled by
provincial governments and are therefore much less expensive.[31]
So, our system would still have ended up being more expensive than the Canadian system.

The Canadian system is not the best system in the world, though it is cheaper than ours. The Canadian system also uses *fee-for-service* payments to doctors, which are a major cause of healthcare inflation and lowered quality.

Conclusion

In addition to the doctors in our system, a majority of whom are being paid on a fee-for-service basis, we also have other private players in the healthcare markets. The type of financial incentives we provide them affects their behavior. The fee-for-service payments to doctors have encouraged a large and powerful drug industry.

The patent system employed for the encouragement of research and development of drugs is further adding to the high cost of drugs. The faulty payment system used in the past for payments to hospitals is responsible for the current high hospital costs. Even having private insurance companies that have to compete with each other for patients and doctors, has the effect of raising the prices of medicine[32] compared to what the prices would be under a single-payer system.

In the next chapter, we discuss some paradoxes that arise in our system and show how they, too, lead to both high costs and inefficiencies.

... the inability of the medical profession to guarantee effectiveness of their treatments has resulted in producing phenomenal income for the doctors. This is just another paradox ...

CHAPTER 4

PARADOXES IN OUR HEALTHCARE SYSTEM

"America's health care system is neither healthy, caring, nor a system." — *Walter Cronkite*

A system based on fee-for-service payments paid to doctors by private insurers not only results in increasing costs, but the resulting incentives affect the behavior of patients, doctors, and other market players in ways that result in paradoxes. The system affects our cultural beliefs about medicine, and the very definition of health. We will first look at the paradoxes resulting from patient behavior.

Patient Behavior

Patients Want to Receive More Care at Higher Prices—a Breakdown of the Law of Supply and Demand

The very fact that we buy insurance from a private company and pay premiums from our pocket might encourage some of us to use more medical services than we actually need. This fact is well known to insurance companies. They even have a name for it: "Moral Hazard."

Though I knew about the phenomenon of Moral Hazard, I never believed that it was a serious problem until I started talking to people about it. I did not want to believe that people would use doctors' services just because they wanted to get something back in return for the insurance premiums they had been paying. But, recent conversations have changed my mind.

I recently talked with an acquaintance who said he had an appointment with his dentist to have his wisdom teeth pulled out. I was a bit surprised, because he was only twenty-five years of age. I asked him if his wisdom teeth were paining? He said that they were not, but he wanted to get them extracted anyway because he knew that one day he would have to do it, so he might as well get them extracted now because he had been paying dental insurance premiums for a long time and had never used dentist's services.

At the time, I found it odd that someone would punish himself unnecessarily so he could reap the benefit from his insurance. I guess he was not thinking about the problems or other complications that might result because of the extraction. But, I now believe this type of attitude is quite common among people who buy health insurance.

Many people view insurance as a necessary evil. They think they can lessen the pain of the payment of insurance premiums by getting something back. They believe if they have been paying into the system for so long then why not make use of the services? Unfortunately, when it comes to healthcare, *getting something back* is not a good idea. Modern medicine always entails some risk to our health. In an attempt to get something back, they can end up hurting themselves.

The Co-Pay Paradox

To partly solve the problem of overuse and abuse of insurance benefits by patients, insurance companies developed the system of co-pays. For each doctor's visit, patients are required to pay a small fixed amount out-of-pocket thus discouraging them from excessive visits to the doctors. In other words, the co-pay protects the patient from the expense of the full doctor's fee while discouraging excessive doctors' visits. Even though the co-pay discourages the number of unnecessary visits to a doctor, it creates another problem.

Consider that you are insured by an insurance company that fixes your co-pay at $20 for each doctor's visit, regardless of the fee the doctor charges. Let us say you develop a medical problem and decide to visit a doctor. If you do not know any doctors in your area, you will have to somehow decide which doctor to visit.

Suppose you find that two doctors in your area might be able to help you. One doctor charges $70 for the visit while the other charges $250 per visit. Since you do not know either of these doctors and your co-pay would be $20 in both cases, you might decide to visit the doctor who charges $250 reasoning that he must be a better doctor since he charges more.

It is easy to see that unlike in true free-markets, the system of co-pay can actually encourage higher prices. It can encourage people to *shop for higher prices* rather than lower ones. This is a breakdown of the law of supply and demand. Many of the problems in our healthcare system are directly or indirectly related to it. Many of the results that the healthcare market is producing are opposite to what we expect in free-markets.

Patients Expect the Doctor to Intervene

One primary care doctor told me that in the early years of his practice, he used to advise his patients on changing their lifestyles or suggest simple home remedies. He thought this would be the best type of treatment for his patients because these were safe treatments, without harmful side effects.

Yet, he remembers the dissatisfaction among some of his patients. Some patients felt that they were not getting much more than what their grandma could give them for free. This scenario is not unusual. Many of us expect doctors to intervene in our sickness. We expect doctors to offer us the types of treatments that only a licensed practitioner is authorized to offer. This may be a prescription for a drug or a procedure that only a licensed physician can perform.

Since we are paying so much money to the doctor, our expectation is that he or she must do for us something that we cannot do ourselves at home—a treatment that only a licensed professional will be able to prescribe or perform. Simple treatments carried out at home might be better for us, but often we are concerned with getting something back from our insurance, and we often put too much trust in modern medicine just because its procedures are more expensive and sound more exotic.

Doctor's Behavior

Not only does our system affect the behavior of patients, it also provides wrong incentives to the doctors for the practice of medicine. It thus affects the doctors' behavior.

Doctors Can Get More Business by Charging More

Just as the co-pay system can encourage patients to choose doctors who charge more, it can also encourage doctors to keep their charges high. Doctors know that under our system of health insurance, patients might prefer to go to doctors who charge more. They know that unless they keep their fees high, some patients will assume that they must not be good doctors. This phenomenon is the opposite of what you would expect in free-markets. It provides a classic example of how the law of supply and demand can break down.

If the law of supply and demand can break down in healthcare markets, you might also expect that so many other things that we take for granted in the free-markets might also not apply in healthcare markets. Such is indeed the case as we will discover in the remaining part of this chapter.

Treatments Based on Drugs and Surgery

Thomas Alva Edison once remarked that the "doctor of the future" will use no medicines. His belief was probably based on his conviction that once the functioning of the human body is better understood, it would be possible to use less risky ways of curing diseases than is possible by the use of drugs. He hoped science would reveal a more thorough understanding of the human body, and it would be possible to reverse the course of diseases through the use of safer natural substances and without the use of drugs that only cure symptoms while causing serious side effects.

It is not known what time-frame Edison had in mind when he used the word "future," but the future he once envisioned has not yet arrived. Medicine has moved in the opposite direction. Even when simple natural cures are possible and diseases can be cured by lifestyle changes, strong medication is usually being prescribed. Edison lived *before the introduction of private insurance* into our healthcare system. He therefore could not have foreseen the impact it could have on the incentives for the practice of medicine, and, therefore, on the development of medicine itself.

Because of the fee-for-service method of payment, and third-party payers, each doctor is essentially a vendor. Unless doctors sell a tangible service, they will not be paid by the insurance companies. Examples of tangible services sold by a doctor and recognized by insurance companies are: prescriptions, tests,and medical procedures.

Advice carries no payment.[33] If a doctor were to advise you on a healthy lifestyle and asked you to pay more attention to your diet, the doctor could have a hard time receiving payment from the insurance company. Moreover, if his or her advice turns out to be valuable, you will not need the doctor to have your prescriptions refilled and the doctor could lose you as a patient.

Thus, the incentive system has made treatment of diseases by drugs and procedures nearly universal. This nearly universal practice, in turn, has convinced us that it must be the only way to treat diseases. Drugs are now considered a necessary part of modern medicine. If we had different incentives in our system and had designed our system in another way, things might have been different.

Suggestions by anyone to cure or treat diseases using natural or non-invasive and safe methods is so uncommon that it strikes as unscientific to most people. What makes these suggestions appear even more unscientific is that they are almost never made by their doctors but usually come from other sources.

More Doctors Do Not Lower the Prices Charged by Doctors or Relieve the Demand for Healthcare (12)

Here is another phenomenon unique to healthcare markets. For those of us accustomed to dealing in free markets, it might seem obvious that to bring down the prices of healthcare, all we have to do is to have more doctors and that would lower the prices the doctors charge.

Having more doctors does not relieve the demand for healthcare. This phenomenon, first observed in 1974 by a Canadian health economist Robert Evans, is called "demand inducement" (12) : *"A personal relationship arises from the significant information differential between physician and patient that permits the physician to exert direct, non-price influence on the demand for his own services."* In other words, doctors can create demand for their own business by making people believe that *they are sicker than they really are.*

Doctors Owning Diagnostic Test Equipment Order More Tests (13)

If you are one of those who believe that doctors always sacrifice their own financial interests to do what is best for their patients then the following should interest you. Studies show that doctors who own their test equipment tend to order more tests (14). Even when doctors order more tests than necessary, they probably do not feel guilty because they know their bill will be paid by the patients' insurance company.

Doctors can also justify the use of more tests by suggesting that they need to protect themselves against malpractice lawsuits. Financial incentives as well as the fear of lawsuits both can conflict with good medicine.

Some states are acutely aware of the problem and have banned doctors from owning test equipment.

Lack of General Practitioners

Another phenomenon, though not directly connected to the free markets, is a consequence of the incentive system for doctors. This is the lack of general practitioners in America. Compared to other countries in the world, America has the least number of general practitioners in proportion to surgeons and other specialists. Although the general practitioners and primary care physicians perform a valuable service, they are not as well paid in the United States as the specialists, who practice riskier and potentially more harmful medicine.

Our system does a great disservice to primary care physicians as well as to the society in general by discouraging the practice of general medicine, while encouraging the practice of surgeries and other risky forms of medicine.

With too many surgeons and not enough primary care physicians, we have a sure-fire recipe for producing too many unnecessary surgeries and not enough people to correctly diagnose and safely treat health problems. This is also a formula to guarantee higher cost of medicine and results in more medical errors, unnecessary deaths, and more malpractice lawsuits.[34]

The High Incomes of U.S. Doctors

Most people attribute the exceptionally high income of doctors to factors such as their ability to save lives or to the long training it takes to become a doctor. Yet, as pointed out in Chapter 1, such factors cannot possibly explain their high income because we are not living in the Soviet Union of the 1950s. Only in the communist Soviet Union of that period were the incomes of various professionals decided by a government body. When determining incomes, the government committees took into account such factors as the contribution made by a profession to society or the number of years required to become a professional. In the United States, it is the markets that determine the income of any given profession. It will be shown below how the faulty markets have benefited doctors.

We will focus on the business model for doctors. One of the reasons why American doctors can earn such high incomes is that the medical profession *cannot guarantee* that treatments prescribed by doctors will be effective in every case. There is neither any way to quantify the benefit provided by a doctor, nor any way to guarantee whether a given treatment will be effective for a particular patient. Only the *probability* of effectiveness of treatments is known.

When a patient walks into a doctor's office, there is an implied understanding that a doctor will do his or her best to help the patient, but *no guarantee of results.* The understanding between the medical profession and society is that doctors will be paid for *trying* to help, rather than for the actual *results* of their treatments.

Historically, doctors have demanded that they be paid for their efforts, regardless of the outcomes. Society has acquiesced. This has resulted in the "fee-for-service" system of payment. Although fee-for-service payments are used in other businesses, in medicine the term has taken on a entirely different meaning: payment for 'services' without regards to 'results.' Thus the term has acquired a very different meaning when used in reference to other businesses, such as auto repair.

Consider auto repair. The mechanics working in a auto repair shop are *expected* to have a complete understanding of the operation of an automobile. If your car is not running, and you take your car to an auto mechanic, you would expect the mechanic to fix your car before you pay the mechanic. It is unlikely you would want to pay just because he or she *tried* to fix it, but failed. However, in the case of doctors, you are expected to pay them, even if they did not heal you, but simply because they *tried.*

Thus, rather than hurting their income, the *inability* of doctors to guarantee the effectiveness of their treatments has actually resulted in an *increase* in their income. This is a paradox. No matter what service a doctor provides, it is paid for, whether it helped the patient or not, or whether it was even needed.

Instead of demanding results (that the doctors cannot guarantee), society has agreed to pay them for their efforts, regardless of the benefit. Whether it is a prescription medication or an expensive surgery costing hundreds of thousands of dollars, the results or benefits are not taken into account when paying doctors. Payments can be *handsome* because they are made by the insurance companies.

Combine the fee-for-service method of payment with the payment from insurance and you have a recipe for very high income. But, that is not all. This method of payment has resulted in incentives that are quite different from what they are for most other businesses.

This results in high incomes for doctors at the expense of quality. Our system rewards bad doctors and punishes the good. How? Consider a doctor in family practice. Since the payment system does not take into account the results, the doctor has no incentive to spend extra time with his or her patients. The doctor will be paid the same amount by the insurance company as long as he or she spends *some* time with the patient, regardless of the duration of the visit or the quality of time spent.

Doctors try to optimize their earnings by packing as many patients into their schedule as possible. Since they will be paid the same whether they spend five minutes or five hours with a patient, it has resulted in doctors reducing their time with each patient to ten-to-fifteen minutes. This time may be enough for a superficial examination of the patient and the writing of a prescription or two, but it is hardly enough to get to the bottom of patients' ailments.

Contrast the situation with that of auto-mechanics. Since they will only be paid if a job is done right, they do not have the luxury of spending only fifteen minutes to fix each car. They must spend as much time as is needed for the repair. They cannot pack in twenty cars in their schedule and expect to be paid for each car just because they *tried* to fix each car whether or not it got fixed.

Thus, the practice of paying doctors for "efforts only" shortchanges patients of their doctor's time and attention, but makes more money for the doctor. Not many doctors seem to feel the need to spend hours with a patient to apprehend a patient's problems. Many of them have not even developed the skills to understand the origins of diseases. Having these types of skills will not enhance their income in this type of a system. So, why bother?

In fact, if a doctor wants to be a good doctor and spend more time with his patients, he or she must see *fewer* patients per day. This will *lower* the doctor's income.

As was indicated previously, drugs are available to deal with most symptoms. They alleviate symptoms, not fundamental problems, and make a doctor's job easier. Doctors do not even need to pick out the right medication the first time. He or she can ask a patient to come to the office again the following week to try another medication if the first one does not work. The insurance provider will pay for each visit.

In this way, the practice of paying doctors for efforts alone has enhanced their incomes over those in careers that must show concrete results. Doctors are paid from the deep pockets of insurance companies and demand large payments by labeling their services as "life-saving." All this adds up to a business model for making huge amounts of money in contrast to professions where concrete results must be produced.

Specialists and surgeons are paid even more than general practitioners for their services because their work involves more risk to the patient. Here the situation is even more egregious and encourages riskier medicine. The result has been even higher income for these doctors and the delivery of more unsafe medicine for patients.

How the Public Perceives the High Income of Doctors: Its Effect on Doctors' Expectations

While the high prices of drugs and other medicine have infuriated the public, the high earnings of doctors have actually helped to add to their prestige. Since most people do not understand the underlying reasons that enable doctors to earn vast sums of money in our system, they associate their high incomes with their ability.

Most Americans have come to regard doctors as superhuman. This also raises the expectation that patients have of their doctors. It is a mixed blessing for both patients and doctors.

While these raised expectations force doctors to live up to their reputation, it can have negative consequences for them, too. Doctors are expected not to miss detecting a disease when a patient comes to them for a checkup. If they do, they risk getting sued. Since detection of diseases can often require judgment, this is an unfair expectation. But judges and juries often side with patients in such cases, since the juries (and judges) have equally high though unjustified expectations of doctors' abilities.

Doctors, in their defense, have taken to ordering extensive and sometimes unnecessary tests. Not only does this give them some protection from lawsuits, but it also adds to their income. This, in turn, has resulted in raising the high cost of medicine even more. An already bad situation is thus being perpetuated.

Caribbean Medical Schools

Because the doctor's business model offers an easy way to make money in the United States, it has attracted the attention of young people starting out in life and searching for a career. This has created a demand for the entry into medical schools. The ease of making money in this profession is what attracts students and increases the competition to get into medical schools.

Entrance into American medical schools is quite competitive and often requires proof of high scholastic achievement. This situation has created an incorrect impression that very high intelligence is required to become a practicing doctor.

However, even lesser-skilled people can make money in the profession. In fact, not too long ago one could enter even excellent medical schools (such as Harvard Medical School) with little more than average grades.

But, entrepreneurs have noticed the ease of making money in the American medical profession. All over the world, and especially in the Caribbean, entrepreneurs have established medical schools for the sole purpose of awarding medical degrees to those denied admission into American medical colleges. These rejected applicants from American medical schools are accepted into these schools with little more than average grades. After graduation, if these graduates can obtain residency in American hospitals and pass the exam for foreign graduates, they can practice in America and make just as much income as American medical graduates.

Medicine is the only profession that offers financial opportunities to all those who can enter the field through the lowering of entry requirements. In other professions, such as law or engineering, a license to practice does not guarantee high income. Consequently, there are no such schools in the Caribbean for professions such as law, engineering, or physics.

Hospitals

Roemer's Law (15)

Roemer's law is little known to the general public but is well known to policymakers in the healthcare field. The law says that when it comes to hospitals, the supply of beds creates its own demand. More succinctly the law states that: *"in an insured population, a hospital bed built is a bed filled."*

Milton Roemer a U.S. Public Health policy expert first articulated the law. His career was full of achievements that spanned several decades. He made several contributions to healthcare policy not only in the United States but also abroad.

For example, he was responsible for launching the first Canadian government-run health insurance program in Saskatchewan.

Roemer was teaching at Cornell in 1961, and at that time he was also examining hospital growth in upstate New York. This was an era of rapid growth in hospital construction in the country. He wanted to know how many hospital beds were needed per thousand people in a given population.

To obtain an answer, Roemer started to keep track of the new beds that were being added to the hospitals at the time. At first he thought that as soon as hospitals had adequate bed capacity, no more beds would be needed. To his dismay, he found that no matter how many beds were added to a hospital, they all seemed to fill up as fast as they were added. It could only mean one thing: doctors were creating demand for the newly added beds.

This was a very troubling implication. However, to the readers of this book, this revelation should not come as a surprise. It is only one more example of how the law of supply and demand breaks down: this time in relation to hospital beds.

'Certificate of Need' (CON) Laws

This observation should have prompted the policymakers to make drastic changes in the healthcare system or even revamp the system. However, in response, they made only a piecemeal change. In 1964 the State of New York passed a "Certificate of Need" law (16).[35] The law required that the state had to grant permission before any new medical facilities could be built.

Subsequently, in 1974, the National Health Planning and Resources Development Act (PL 93-641) imposed similar requirements on states. This federal legislation mandated that all U.S. states have a "Certificate of Need (CON)" requirement similar to that of New York or they could be denied federal funding. Though the act was subsequently repealed in 1980s under President Reagan's administration, despite the removal of the federal requirement, certificate of need laws currently exist in nearly two-thirds of the states.

Yet, *certificate of need laws do nothing to solve the underlying causes as to why unnecessary medicine is being dispensed* in the first place. Limiting the number of hospitals to reduce unnecessary care is like trying to reduce bank robberies in a city by reducing the number of banks in the city rather than by catching the robbers.

Hospitals that Own More Equipment Tend to be the Costliest

Dartmouth University conducted a study some time ago to find out which hospitals use the most expensive equipment to treat their patients.[36] The study found that the equipment used by a hospital is not dependent upon the needs of the population. In the same geographical area and in the same population, they found that the hospitals that had the most expensive equipment tended to use it the most often.

Once again, it is not the needs of the patients that are getting priority but the financial gain of the hospitals and doctors. Hospitals, in turn, acquire equipment to please the doctors. The more equipment the hospital has, the more appealing it is to the doctors to be associated with it. In other words, money appeal to the doctors ultimately results in higher costs for the patients.

Hospitals with More Equipment Become Less Affordable for the Poor

If healthcare markets worked like free-markets, you would expect the hospitals to buy only the necessary equipment. If a hospital bought too many high tech machines, it would be a bad investment and the hospital could lose money because of injudicious spending. But, nothing of the sort occurs in the healthcare markets. In these markets, when hospitals invest in unnecessary expensive equipment, they easily recoup their investment. They do that by overusing equipment on patients who do not need it as well as by keeping their prices high since they know that their insured patients do not care about prices. *These high prices make testing out of reach for patients not covered by insurance and who would like to pay out-of-pocket.*

Studies by the Physician Payment Review Commission (PPRC) and the Government Accountability Office (GAO) show that because we have too many mammography machines, prices are set to double over what they should be because these machines are being underutilized. *In other words, too much monetary investment is making care unaffordable for many.* Such paradoxes can occur only in a poorly designed system such as ours.

Premature Discharge of Patients from Hospitals

I was once talking to a woman who said she was pregnant and wanted to stay in the hospital for a little longer after she had given birth to her baby daughter. But, the hospital would not let her stay even though she thought she was not healthy enough to be released. Eventually, she came home and had to take a long leave from her job to recuperate. She did not know that her situation was not unique. It was the result of incentives involved in the payment system for hospitals.

Currently, as was mentioned previously, hospitals are paid on a Diagnostic Related Group (DRG) system. Under this plan, a hospital receives a lump-sum payment based on whatever diagnosis the physician makes.

For example, there is a fixed payment for pregnancy. It does not matter how many days the mother stays in the hospital, the insurance company will pay only a fixed amount to the hospital. In such cases, it is against the interest of the hospital to allow patients to stay any longer than absolutely necessary. In such a system there will always be some patients who will be discharged from the hospital early whether they are ready for it or not. Thus, even though the DRG system controls costs, the needs of some of the patients are being sacrificed.

Drug Companies

Consequences of Marketing Tactics of Drug Companies

In Chapter 3, we discussed how the patent system for drug development affects the costs of drugs. This chapter will discuss how subtle sales techniques used by drug companies are changing society's belief about *health, disease, and prevention.*

Drug companies have a need to be subtle in the sales of their products. They must be able to convince patients that their products are *solely* for the good of their patients and the companies must be able to disguise any financial motives. One way for them to do this is to cultivate a society that believes in the need for their products and then plant seeds about the benefits of specific products.

In addition, drug companies need the help of doctors to market their product. Enlisting the help of doctors is relatively easy. The incentives of drug companies and doctors are aligned, and doctors also benefit from the sale of more prescription drugs. Both doctors and drug companies also benefit from suppressing the use of safer natural and easily available products. As a result of the drug marketing techniques, *medical advice as well as medical education have been affected* as are American *society's beliefs* about heath and disease prevention. Let us see how.

Prevention through Drugs

'You need us to avoid us' – Medical Profession to Patients

A good diet, exercise, and healthy lifestyle ought to be the mainstay of any prevention program. The very reason for preventing a disease is to be able to avoid drugs and other forms of medical interventions. Unfortunately, doctors, drug companies, and the medical profession have turned the whole idea of prevention on its head. Doctors often suggest the use of drugs to *slightly* lower the risk of a *possible* future disease without mentioning the serious side effects of these drugs. The harmful side effects of drugs often result in more serious problems than the ones they prevent. The reason for suggesting drugs for prevention is simple: prescribing drugs *makes money* for the doctors and the drug companies whereas prevention without drugs *does not.*

The widespread use of statins is a good example of the overuse of drugs. These cholesterol-lowering drugs are often given to patients with high cholesterol levels. However statins can have serious side effects including swelling of muscles and damage to the kidney and liver. The same drug that is peddled for heart health[37] can end up weakening the heart (17).

Inventing New Diseases for the Healthy; Ignoring Those Truly in Need

There are more healthy people in the world than sick people. Healthy people, therefore, form a *larger* market than the market comprised of sick people. Therefore, financially, it makes sense to develop drugs for the *larger* market--people who are otherwise healthy but might suffer from minor symptoms related to a less than perfect lifestyle. The result is that today there are more medications for people who are healthy and who do not really need them and not as many for those who are seriously sick and need them the most.[38]

If recently you have come across names of some new diseases that you had not heard of before, you are not alone. Several years ago there were no diseases such as Attention Deficit Disorder (ADD), Social Anxiety Disorder (SAD), Seasonal Adjustment Disorder (SAD), Post-Menopausal Syndrome (PMS), Pre-menstrual Syndrome (PMS), GERD or Acid Reflux.

These diseases are popularized by drug companies for the purposes of expanding the market for their drugs. In our busy lifestyle, any of us can suffer minor symptoms, related to normal life stresses and develop some of the symptoms associated with the above diseases. These symptoms are often not serious and can be viewed as minor discomforts of life. But, drug companies and doctors have convinced the public that these must be viewed as serious diseases and medications must be taken for their treatment.

Also, changes in body that are the result of normal aging have been characterized as diseases. One such example is the *post-menopausal syndrome*. Over last several decades, millions of women have been urged to take hormones to avert symptoms of post-menopausal syndrome. What is not mentioned to the patients is that serious side effects can occur including an increased risk of cancer.[39] In many cases, such therapies can turn out to be worse than the disease they were intended to treat.

Tinkering with Nutritional and Medical Science

You might have noticed that advice in the areas of food and health keeps changing from year to year. For example, a few decades ago we were told that saccharine, a sugar substitute, was good for us. Today, we are being warned that it might be a carcinogen. Margarine was touted as good for us because that way we could avoid eating saturated fat. Today, we are told it contains *trans-fat*, one of the worst type of fats to consume. Only a few years ago, coffee was bad for you. Today we are told it can be good for you. Many years ago, tonsillectomies were performed routinely on children. Today, we are told that they might not be appropriate.

Examples of changing advice abound in food and medicine. We can never be sure if what we are being told today will turn out to be false tomorrow. In fact, we could be hurting ourselves by following medical or food advice. If we had followed food advice several years ago and used saccharine as a sweetener, we would have increased our risk of getting cancer. Use of aspartame would have increased our risk of neurological diseases (18).

Why is it that in the areas of natural sciences such as in physics and chemistry, the information does not change from year to year like it does in the area of healthcare and nutrition? Newton's laws are still as true as they were three centuries ago. The reason is simple: *the information on diet and health is heavily influenced by the financial interests of food and medicine industries.*

If the only way the food, drug, and medical industries tried to achieve their goals was to use the methods employed by manufacturers of other consumer products, things would not be so bad. However, drug companies have decided that a more effective way to market their products is to *influence medical education itself.* Instead of being a quest for truth, *science has become a valuable tool for marketing.* Drug companies have found a way to influence medical community by ghostwriting articles favorable to their products in medical and scientific journals published under the names of doctors and other medical researchers. *In this way, doctors and drug companies have become equal partners in fraud.*

Examples of such interference in scientific literature abound. For example, in response to a recent lawsuit, documents were unsealed in a court testimony, which showed that GlaxoSmith-Kline was paying doctors to ghostwrite articles in medical journals (19) on behalf of other doctors. *Of course, all this can happen only with the blessing of the unethical doctors and researchers who gain recognition by getting published in the prestigious medical journals* whereas drug companies benefit by the publication of favorable information about their drugs.

Once the information is published in the prestigious medical journals, *this information gets passed on into the medical textbooks.* At this level, it is taught by professors in medical schools to the next generation of medical students. The information in medical books and taught by the professors is taken to be hard science. *Once the students become practicing doctors, they will believe and practice what they have learned in medical school.* They reject information that comes from *any other source and which conflicts with their medical school education.*

The very soul of science can be tinkered with by using these practices. Science can be reduced to a marketing tool for the profit of companies. The biggest tragedy is that *society pays the ultimate price.*

Medical journals, however, are not the only information sources that are influenced by drug companies. Even medical textbooks cannot be trusted. For example, a medical-school psychiatry textbook published in 1999 listed as co-authors the chairs of Emory University and Stanford University, but the book was actually ghostwritten by GlaxoSmithKline (20).

Detailed discussions of how the drug companies use various techniques and methods for sale of their products and influence beliefs of society are available in some excellent books such as that by Marcia Angell's *The Truth About the Drug Companies:*

How They Deceive Us and What to do about it. Her book
recounts the various strategies that are routinely employed by
drug companies for the sale of drugs (21). Angell served as the
editor of the *New England Journal of Medicine* for
approximately two decades and was in a position to understand
the intricacies of the sales methods employed by the drug
industry. Another excellent book is *Anatomy of an Epidemic:
Magic Bullets, Psychiatric Drugs, and the Astonishing Rise of
Mental Illness in America* by Robert Whitaker, which focuses
on how the psychiatric drugs are being oversold in America
(22).

Another good book written by Joseph Dumit, Professor of
Anthropology at University of California—Davis, is *Drugs for
Life: How Pharmaceutical Companies Define Our Health*
(23). It provides an anthropologist's perspective on how the
core social beliefs about our health can be influenced by drug
companies.

Cure versus Treatment

Have you noticed that the use of the word 'cure' has almost
disappeared from the medical language? Whenever doctors
and drug companies talk about a disease, they mostly talk
about 'treating' the disease not 'curing' it. In the last few
decades, our drug industry has developed many drugs to treat
diseases and very few to cure any disease. Although the fee-
for-service medicine has been practiced in this country for a
long time, this change has occurred mainly in in the recent
decades. In the early part of the twentieth century, drugs were
developed, and research was carried out with the intent to cure
diseases. For example, antibiotics were developed that truly

cured patients by killing the germs.

Also, many diseases were cured by supplying the missing nutrients in the diet. For example, diseases such as beriberi, scurvy, rickets, and iron deficiency anemia were all found to be curable by supplying essential nutrients. The cures turned out to be simple, inexpensive, and effective. It was a matter of supplying the missing nutrients through consumption of foods.

For example, beriberi was cured by supplying unpolished rice. Scurvy was easily cured by having its victims eat oranges (24). And iron deficiency anemia could be cured simply by leaving water overnight in an iron bucket and having the patient drink the water in the morning. Rickets could be prevented by taking cod liver oil.

However, few such cures have been developed since the 1950s. Exact reasons for this state of affairs are difficult to determine. It is quite possible that all the diseases that were caused by simple nutritional deficiencies have been discovered. But, it could also be that there are no financial incentives for developing cures. Treatments make more money than cures.

Drug companies as well as doctors like chronic illnesses. If a cure were found, they would cease to be chronic. Chronic diseases make maximum profits for the drug companies. These are *also* the diseases that cost the patient, their insurance company, and the country a lot of money. Type 2 diabetes happens to be one of the costliest diseases in the United States. It, thus, makes a lot of money for the medical profession. In many cases (25), this disease is believed to be completely curable by diet and exercise. But the medical profession has incentives to perpetuate its current status as a chronic disease and dole out prescription medications rather than treating it as a lifestyle disease, which in many cases it is.

Since drug companies work on a profit motive and potential profits are huge, it should come as no surprise that they would employ all efforts to maximize their profits, whether or not these are totally ethical. However, *ultimately it is our policies that provide incentives to the drug companies to conduct the business as they do.*

Ultimately it is us–society and the politicians, who are to blame for allowing these policies to exist and to encourage the behavior that stems from these policies. If we blame drug companies for everything, we will be like the person who allows the fox to guard his henhouse and then blames the fox when he eats some of the chickens.

A later chapter shows how we can change incentives in order to change the behavior of drug companies and other medical providers.

Influence of the System on our Everyday Beliefs about Health

Some beliefs about health have become ingrained in the minds of most Americans. Many Americans believe that regular checkups and regular visits to a medical professional are necessary to stay healthy. These include practices such as regular visits to a dentist, regular health checkups, wisdom tooth removal, tonsillectomies, regular prostate checkups, regular mammograms, and so forth. We rarely pay attention to where these beliefs might have *originated*.[40]Although these practices appeal to our commonsense, a deeper investigation shows that many of these practices can be harmful to our health.[41]

The medical profession makes these recommendations motivated by its financial interests. But such recommendations also have a profound influence on our understanding about *health, sickness, and prevention*. The main message being conveyed to the society is that people need medical intervention *today* to prevent *possible* medical interventions in the *future*. In other words, society is being sold the idea that there is no way to avoid medical intervention. This view is necessarily false. In reality, people in many societies in the world live long lives without any modern medical interventions.[42]

Visit your Dentist Regularly

Most Americans believe that somehow it is impossible to maintain healthy teeth unless one makes regular visits to a dentist. They forget that not too long ago there were no dentists and people still had healthy teeth. This fact was first brought to light by Dr. Weston Price,[43] (1870-1948), a Cleveland dentist. He visited Switzerland and other countries of the world to investigate dental care in different parts of the world. He observed that among certain tribes of Switzerland there were no dentists; yet, people had much healthier teeth than they did in America.

Even today in some developing nations in the world, people rarely visit dentists. This shows that it is possible to have healthy teeth all your life without medical help. Prevention of dental problems is easy. Through simple brushing and flossing and maintenance of good general health, it should be possible to have healthy teeth for life without the need to go to a dentist.

I can say this with confidence, because I have had only one dental visit in my whole life. There are certain habits that are simple (but are not generally known) that can help anyone reduce or eliminate the need for seeing a dentist. I grew up in a culture where as a child, I was taught to go to the bathroom after every meal and rinse out my mouth after eating. This was also a custom in our extended family and among my relatives. If any guests came to our home, they would routinely be shown the bathroom after dinner. When I went to eat with my relatives, they treated me the same way.

Yet, after migrating to America and adopting the lifestyle here, I gave up on some of my habits for a number of years. I started to develop occasional mild pains in my teeth. At this point, I decided to go to a dentist. Not that the pains were intense enough to warrant a visit to a dentist, but I wanted to visit a dentist *anyway* because some of my friends used to chide me for not knowing what a dentist's office looked like.

So, I decided to visit a dentist to see what goes on in a dentist's office. I made an appointment with a dentist near my house. My dentist was genuinely surprised that I had good teeth at my age without ever having visited a dentist before. He did not find much wrong with my teeth, but I asked him to clean my teeth anyway. I guess that satisfied my curiosity and I have resumed my childhood practice of rinsing my teeth after every meal. It has now been another twenty years, and I have not had the need to visit a dentist again.

Take your Medications Regularly

Mothers often tell their children to take medications regularly or they will not get well. It is a sure way to ingrain in their minds that use of drugs is inevitable for health. While medicines might be necessary in some situations, such teachings given to us at an early age can become a part of our belief system and can remain with us even when we grow up. Not all of us are always aware that medications can cause harm too. Even in our adult life, we might assume that medications are always good for us and are the only way to heal.

Must You Get Physical Checkups Every Year?

Many misunderstandings about health and healthcare are based on the belief that medicine is an exact science–just like physics or chemistry. People make the mistake of believing that the human body is as well understood as an automobile (for example). Just as a well-designed car can run longer and better by good preventive maintenance performed by a mechanic, they believe so can our body function better if we allow it to be checked by a healthcare professional and get it regularly treated.

But there are many differences between cars and the human body. Cars are man-made machines.Therefore, mechanics have much better understanding of the workings of cars than doctors have of the human body. Moreover when we take our car to a dealership to get it repaired, we know to be skeptical because the mechanic might want to fix things in our car that may not need fixing. With doctors, the same caution should apply. Yet, many of us put greater faith in doctors even though the workings of human body are less well understood and the doctors operate under perverse system of incentives.

While it might be acceptable to get regular checkups if you stop there. But often there is more to these checkups. After the checkups, your doctor will usually also recommend medicine to reduce the risk of your getting a disease in the *future*. For example, high blood pressure or high cholesterol levels are not diseases in themselves. They are only risk factors.They might or might not cause disease in the future. But doctors often prescribe medications to reduce the numbers.

All prescriptions medications have a potential for harm (that is why they require a prescription). In addition, almost all drugs stress out your liver and kidneys.[44] If you know about safer alternatives to modern allopathic medicine, it might be all right for you to get regular checkups, but, in many cases in the long run, the checkups and the follow-up treatments that are recommended can be harmful.[45]

In addition, some types of testing can require the use of imaging techniques such as X-rays, CAT scans, or PET scans. These imaging techniques can expose the body to harmful radiation that has proven cancer-causing effects.[46]

When during the healthcare debate of 2009, President Barack Obama mentioned that it is not recommended for younger women to get regular screenings for breast cancer, an uproar ensued against what he said. People mistrusted him as if it were an attempt to infringe upon their freedom so that government could save money. But consider the following facts about mammograms. First of all, mammograms involve subjecting the patient to radiation. There is some risk that the radiation itself will cause the cancer that it is supposed to detect.

In addition, the interpretation of mammograms is subject to question. It is possible to get false positives or false negatives. The tests with younger women are harder to interpret. Under such a scenario, it might be better not to have oneself tested often. It makes much more sense to use preventive care but not have frequent mammograms. It might be far better to make liberal use of fruits and vegetables and other antioxidants and avoid known carcinogens, such as alcohol and tobacco, that increase the rate of breast cancer.

But invariably when suggestions such as those made by President Obama (or other government officials) conflict with those made by private providers, people seem to be less skeptical about the motives of the healthcare professionals (who might be inducing you into using more services because of the profit motive) and more skeptical about the government that might be trying to save money. Thus sound advice can often be mistrusted by the public and unsound advice easily believed.

Conclusion

The incentive system not only affects the prices and quality of medicine but also our understanding about disease prevention and health in general. In a later chapter, we will discuss what we can do to reform the system.

But first in the next chapter, we analyze the various proposals that politicians have made to reform the healthcare system and we examine whether these proposals have the potential to solve long-term healthcare problems.

In 2009, the national healthcare debate had taken on the atmosphere of a dinner mystery theater with everyone trying to pick out a villain....Health insurance companies are disliked by many. Therefore, those who picked them for a villain did not feel the need to explain or even understand their role in raising prices...

Yes, insurance is a problem. But not in the way most lawmakers perceived it to be. Insurance company profit margins are not the problem. The problem is that we have created a system that in order to function requires the existence of health insurance companies.

CHAPTER 5

WHY THE POPULAR REFORM PROPOSALS WILL NOT FIX HEALTHCARE

In September 2009, President Barack Obama presented his healthcare proposal to the Congress, which for the first time in the nation's history, promised coverage to everyone in the country under some form of a insurance plan, regardless of the individual's health or income. It was called the Patient Protection and Affordable Care Act (ACA). It promised to cover everyone while keeping the incentives for the healthcare providers mostly *unchanged*.

Even though the President's plan did not make structural changes in the way the healthcare was to be paid for and did not threaten to cut the profits to the healthcare providers, it met with intense opposition. In response to this proposal, legislators offered a number of alternative reform proposals. Most of these were not entirely new and had been suggested many times even before the President's proposal.

Although the Affordable Care Act has now passed, it is unlikely to solve all our problems. As of this writing, unanticipated problems associated with the law have cropped up. Insurance premiums are rising faster than ever, and private companies are cutting work hours of employees to get around the provisions of the law that require the companies to buy health insurance for their full-time employees.

All this would mean more financial burden on the government. Although the law contains some cost-cutting measures, it now appears that the law as enacted might unduly strain the federal budget. It is, therefore, very likely that some of the proposals that were suggested earlier during the healthcare debate would be suggested again.

We will now examine if these reform proposals and alternative suggestions that have been suggested, have any merit. Had any of these proposals been enacted, could they have solved our healthcare problems?

Although most proposals were aimed at solving the cost problem, others were aimed at the quality problem. Suggestions were also aimed at changing the legal system to limit malpractice suits *without examining why so many lawsuits occur*, and whether limiting damages for doctors would actually reduce medical costs for the public.

Many proposals were aimed at improving the insurance industry *without presenting any evidence that profits of insurance companies are raising underlying healthcare costs*. Some reform proposals even suggested partially undoing the protection of insurance, by making patients more responsible financially for their healthcare by expansion of health savings accounts.

Almost no suggestions were made for changing the hospital system although the *hospital costs comprise the single biggest item in most healthcare bills.* Almost no suggestions were made to change the incentives of the doctors although they control the delivery of medicine. Almost no attention was given to drug costs except perhaps making it easy for drug companies to obtain patents or allowing Americans to buy drugs from abroad.[47]

When the Affordable Care Act eventually passed, none of these proposals got enacted into law. Even though these proposals provided good ideas, these proposals would not have solved the long-term cost problems.

Some of the proposals might have brought down the cost of healthcare in the short run, but would not have done much for the long-term cost increases. It is the accelerating cost of healthcare as illustrated by the hockey-stick curve shown in Chapter 2, that is the problem. Unless something is done to change the system, which is responsible for the shape of the cost curve of Chapter 2, the long-term costs will not be controlled.

Who is the Villain in the Healthcare System?

I vividly remember the mood in the country after President Obama unveiled his healthcare proposal in the September of 2009. The national healthcare debate had taken on the atmosphere of a dinner mystery theater with everyone trying to pick out a villain. Among the cast of characters were the usual suspects: the doctors, the hospitals, the drug companies, insurance companies, malpractice lawsuits, and the government.

To most Republicans, the government, insurance companies, and the medical malpractice suits were the villains. To most

Democrats, the insurance companies or drug companies were the villains. Insurance companies were picked out by the lawmakers on both sides. Neither side presented any solid evidence that excessive profits by insurance companies were responsible for rising healthcare costs. Health insurance companies are disliked by many Americans. Therefore, those who picked them for a villain did not feel the need to explain or even understand their role in raising prices.

Solutions were then designed to correct the behavior of their favorite villain–the insurance companies. Most solutions focused on modifying the behavior of this villain. Surprisingly, few suggested eliminating their existence altogether. Most of the solutions focused on the insurance industry even though this industry is not truly a part of the healthcare industry.[48]

The question that the lawmakers failed to ask was–will making the insurance companies more efficient automatically rein in the *underlying* medical costs? As discussed earlier in Chapter 1, *all* the players in our healthcare system (doctors, hospitals, and drug companies) charge several times what their counterparts do in other countries. Don't we need to worry about these costs too, if we have to reform the system?

These underlying costs are truly the problem. No insurance company can possibly provide coverage at low cost until the underlying costs are checked. No solution focused on this critical issue.

The Elephant in the Room

In picking out the villain every lawmaker ignored the *elephant in the room*–the healthcare *system* itself. Remember what we have already discussed in Chapter 2, the two elements of this system that are most responsible for runaway costs of medicine are the following:

1. The key feature of our system: paying for medicine through insurance

   and

2. The practice of paying doctors for their *services* rather than *results*. We also make higher payments for unsafe medicine.

Yes, *insurance is a problem* but not in the way most lawmakers perceive it to be. The *problem* is that we have created a system that in order to function *requires the existence of health insurance companies*.

If we want to solve our cost problems, *we might have to demolish the whole system that depends on payments through insurance*. But none of the suggestions made by law makers was to eliminate insurance altogether from the healthcare system. Their suggestions were to *keep insurance in the system* but to make it more efficient.

The lawmakers were right to assume that the insurance companies *cannot* be expected to act more selflessly simply because we want them to. Laws would have to be passed to force them to. But they failed to note that there are *other players* in the market too. The behavior of these players is also affecting the functioning of the markets.

All players in the system are acting according to the incentives provided by the system. Patients are demanding more medicine because they think they have paid premiums to insurance companies and should get back as much as possible from their years of payment into the system. Doctors are performing more procedures and more risky ones because *that is where the money is*. Insurance companies are no exception. They are trying to make profits by charging higher premiums as well as by denying benefits when they can.

But remember, while the enrollees want insurance companies to be generous, the stockholders want profits. Company CEOs are stuck between a rock and a hard place. They must be fair to the enrollees and also be able to answer to their shareholders who only care for profits.

Moral Behavior Solution

Some people think that everything in our system would work out well if only all the players in the system acted more *morally*. This is an unreasonable expectation, at best. Sure, if everybody in the world were totally moral, the world would be a wonderful place. We would not have to pay attention to the design of our healthcare system, or economic system or political system. Any system would work well.

Unfortunately, the world is not a selfless place. As long as the incentives in our system are what they are, the players will keep on acting as they are. As long as the music is playing, dancers will keep on dancing. If we want the dancers to dance a different dance, we must change the music.

We do not want a type of system that requires doctors, drug companies, hospitals, and other players in the game to be selfless in order for the system to succeed. We want a system that will succeed despite their selfishness.

Capitalism works not because people are unselfish. It works because people are selfish, but capitalism transforms their selfish behavior through the magic of well-designed markets so that it ends up benefiting the whole society. Let's remember the words of Adam Smith.

It is not from the benevolence of the butcher, the brewer, or the baker that we expect our dinner, but from their regard to their own self-interest. We address ourselves not to their humanity but to their self-love.... — Adam Smith, *An Inquiry into the Nature and Causes of the Wealth of Nations.*

How then do we change the game plan and get different results? This question will be addressed in Chapter 6. For now, let us examine what has been proposed and see why most reform proposals fall short of the goal.

Suggested Reforms in the Insurance Industry

Allowing Insurance Companies to Sell Insurance Across State Lines

A main suggestion coming from the political right has been to allow health insurance companies to sell insurance across state lines.

During his presidential bid of 2008, Senator John McCain, in addition to other suggestions, echoed his party's position and emphasized the idea that allowing companies to sell insurance across state lines would result in a major lowering of healthcare prices. The premise behind the suggestion was that the high prices charged by doctors, hospitals, and drug companies were somehow not the problem. Like many, he saw the real problem as the profit gouging by the insurance companies. He argued, that if there was more competition among the insurance companies, they would charge less and profits and healthcare costs would come down.

However, his analysis missed a few points. Not only was his strategy *not going to bring down underlying medical costs,* but it was unlikely to reform even the insurance industry. It is true that if the selling of insurance across the state lines is permitted, then there will be more competition among the insurance companies for a short time, driving the less-efficient companies out of business. But he failed to note that the strategy would work only for the first few years after its implementation until the most-inefficient insurance companies were driven out of business. After a few years, we would be left with a smaller number of national companies and reduced competition. Because of this reduced competition, the companies could again afford to be less efficient.

Basically, we would be back to square one. Insurance companies are not like manufacturing companies that thrive on manufacturing efficiency. They do not create value. They are in the business of redistributing money by collecting it from a mixed population of healthy and sick and giving it to the sick. If they cannot make ends meet, they only have two ways to survive: either increase premiums or deny benefits. Each company would choose according to its business strategy, but neither of these choices is likely to be good for the consumers.

Moreover, if companies are allowed to do business across state lines, companies will establish their headquarters in the states where the standards are lax and where they can easily deny paying for certain types of care. It is a very risky proposition, indeed, to entrust something as important as healthcare to lax standards.

In the best case scenario, even if we are able to improve the situation by enacting laws to overcome some of these shortcomings, we would not have accomplished our goal to contain the *underlying runaway medical costs*. All we would have accomplished is to reform the insurance industry. Most of our efforts would be in vain.

Purchasing Co-Ops

Another strategy often promoted by some politicians also focuses on the insurance industry. They suggest that it would be better to form large purchasing cooperatives by bringing together large number of people to form groups with increased buying power. The idea was prompted by observation of group insurance plans, which employers often offer to employees.

Most Americans already buy their insurance through their employers and are in employment-based groups. Large employers pay low premiums. Some observers, therefore, have concluded that perhaps it is the wholesale purchasing power of large groups that is responsible for the lower premiums.

However, this conclusion misses important facts. First, the reason insurance companies are willing to sell insurance to employee groups is because *employed* workers are generally *healthy*. It is *health status* of the group that brings down their risk—not the size of the group. Insurance companies are willing to insure employee groups even without knowing the complete health status of the individuals within the group because employed people are generally healthier than the rest of the population. Even if employees in this group fall *seriously* ill, they will very likely lose their job and thus eventually lose insurance benefits. These type of considerations make these groups less risky for insurance companies.

The size of a group is not the sole determiner of the risk. The health status of the individuals in the group is much more important. If the group is large but consists mostly of sick individuals, no insurance company can afford to offer lower rates. Only employer groups formed from large numbers of healthy workers is where the idea works.

If we tried to make the idea work by forming groups of homogeneous populations consisting of roughly the same proportion of healthy and sick in each group, the most we could accomplish would be to make our health insurance industry fairer and more competitive. But, we still have not solved the problem of *underlying runaway medical costs.*

Less Regulation of Insurance Companies Over the Type of Coverage They Offer

Some people feel that if there was less regulation over insurance companies over the types of coverage they offer, more insurance products will be on the market. Thus people will have more choices to pick a product that suits their needs. They believe in this way, lower-cost products can be provided by the insurance companies. However, less regulation over insurance companies is not a good idea. Because it also provides an opportunity for the companies to offer products that might appear attractive to consumers when they are healthy, but might not be adequate when they are sick and need coverage. At that time, it will be too late for consumers to do anything about it.

We buy insurance for our peace of mind. Those of us who have never been seriously ill have no accurate estimate of the costs of our very expensive healthcare system or other problems in our system that builds fortunes for the healthcare providers from the misfortunes of the sick. When we are sick, it will be the wrong time to find out. Everyone needs assurance that when the catastrophe strikes, they will be covered. Regulations are needed to ensure that *catastrophic needs are covered*. Less regulation in this important area opens the door for the rip-off artists who promise but do not deliver. If we allow this to happen, it can cause even more nightmares for the sick and needy.

Tax Incentives for People to Shop for Their Own Insurance

In July of 2001, Dr. Milton Friedman published an article (26) in which he pointed out that government provides tax breaks to employers for providing healthcare as one of the fringe benefits of employment. On the other hand, individuals who buy health insurance on their own get no such tax break. Not only is the playing field tilted against the individual buyer, but even those who get their health insurance from the employer do not necessarily get the type of insurance best suited to their needs.

Dr. Friedman thought it would be better to allow individual employees to shop for insurance on their own but level the playing field for all. This could be done by either by taking away the tax advantaged status of the employers or giving same tax advantages to individuals who buy insurance on their own. This also might encourage insurance companies to offer more products suitable for a greater number of individuals. Ever since the paper was published, many politicians on the right have caught on to the idea and have offered this suggestion as part of their reform package for healthcare. Most believe that the playing field should be leveled.

While Dr. Friedman's suggestion can certainly provide more choice in buying insurance, *it also does nothing to reduce underlying medical costs.* There are other problems with the proposal as well. If you are healthy, you do stand to save money because you may choose from plans designed for the healthy. On the other hand, if you are healthy enough to work but have a medical condition, you might have to pay a lot more for your insurance because you would likely lose the price protection that comes from being in a group plan.

Since Dr. Friedman's proposal was made many years before the passage of Affordable Care Act, many people with pre-existing conditions would have had difficulty buying an individual policy. Dr. Friedman also failed to note that large employers often contract with several insurance companies and do offer choices to their employees about buying into different plans.

Public Option

The public option was a hot topic during the healthcare debate in 2009. President Barack Obama had promoted the idea of a public option. The plan was for the federal government to become one of the insurers in the marketplace and offer insurance just like any other private insurers thus competing with them. Many people thought that government-backed insurance would be trusted more than that coming from private insurers.

Such a federal insurance organization would have no need to earn profits; thus, it could offer lower premiums. Since it would not have a profit motive, it would not have to deny benefits when patients were in critical need. Thus, it was also likely to become the largest insurer with the greatest bargaining power with the providers of healthcare.

The possibility that government could become the insurance of choice for the vast majority of the population was threatening to the private insurance industry. Because of pressure from this industry, the idea of a public option was eventually defeated in the congress.

Even if the public option had succeeded, our problems would not have been solved. Currently, government is the insurer of people on Medicare and Medicaid, but still the medical costs have not been contained. This is so because we were hoping to produce lower costs in medicine by reforming the insurance industry, *rather than focusing on underlying medical costs.*

Electronic Medical Records (EMRs)

Promise of Improvement in Quality and Cost

The Institute of Medicine (IOM) is a part of the National Academy of Sciences (NAS), a private nonprofit organization. It was established in 1970 to advise the government in the areas of medical care, research, and education. In its important report, *To Err is Human* (27) issued in 2000, it mentioned that between 44,000 and 98,000 people die unnecessarily in American hospitals from problems that are quite preventable. This report caused quite a stir among health policy experts.

To improve the quality problems noted in its first report, the Institutes of Medicine issued a second report in March of 2001, *Crossing the Quality Chasm* (28). This second report pointed out that one of the problems with the healthcare system was its fragmentation which results in duplication of certain services and tests. The lack of access to information results in delays or errors, which can cause injury or death in certain emergency situations.

The report suggested that one of the ways to improve the situation was to have a more streamlined system created through electronic medical records, which would be accessible to medical providers as patients moved within the system. This would eliminate the need for duplicate tests. By providing timely information to the providers, it might possibly save lives in emergencies.

In his *Affordable Care Act*, President Obama made electronic medical records one of the priorities. As a part of the stimulus package that was passed to help the country out of the deep recession that occurred at the end of the year 2008, President Obama allocated funds to doctors and hospitals for the conversion of paper records into electronic medical records.

Impact of Electronic Medical Records on the Quality of Healthcare

The process of converting paper records into electronic medical records has just started and will probably take a few more years to be fully implemented. It remains to be seen how much benefit this strategy yields. I believe that at first, the electronic records are likely to be a mixed bag. While the electronic records provide easy access to the data, readily available data is useful, only if it is *accurate*. If incorrect data is accidentally entered into the records, it could cause more harm than good.

As an example, a recent implementation of EMRs at the Children's Hospital of Pittsburgh (CHP) unexpectedly resulted in adverse outcomes. After conversion to Electronic records, it was discovered that the mortality rate there more than doubled (29).

It is possible that after the kinks in the system are worked out, the system with electronic records will work better than the one we have now.[49] Yet, to insure the accuracy of these records, *patient input* would be required. There would have to be some provision that allows patients to keep an eye on what is in their medical records so they can readily correct any errors if they spot them. No one in the system stands to lose as much from the incorrect entry into the records as do the patients themselves.

Disadvantages of Electronic Medical Records

Sticky Diagnoses and Second Opinions

Diagnoses made by doctors are not always correct. Some diseases and conditions have a pathological basis and can be determined with certainty using tests. Other diagnoses are based on the *judgment* of the doctor. A doctor's judgment can be *wrong*.

If doctors see patients and want to get paid by the insurance company, they might be required to *name* a disease on the insurance form. In other words, even if the doctors are not sure of the diagnosis, they might be inclined to fill out the form using their best guess. Therein lies the shortcoming of our system. Not all diseases have a confirmatory test; yet, the insurance companies might expect that diseases are named on the claim forms.[50] This is one of the less talked about shortcomings of our third-party payment system.

Under the system of paper records, a patient could go to another doctor and ask for another independent opinion. If the second doctor had not seen the first diagnosis maybe the second doctor would be able to make a new and possibly more accurate diagnosis. However, if the second doctor has instantaneous access via electronic records to the diagnosis already made by the first doctor, he or she might be reluctant to change the diagnosis that has already been made. A wrong diagnosis coupled with a treatment with drugs or other risky procedures is a recipe for guaranteed harm.

Effect of Electronic Medical Records on Cost

While electronic medical records do have the potential of decreasing medical errors (if they are kept accurate and up to date), some people have also recommended their use for lowering the medical costs.

Electronic medical records do have the potential to save costs, by eliminating the need for duplicate tests and saving on administrative costs. But, this effect is rather small. One study estimated that by switching to the electronic medical records, we can save 6 percent of administrative costs (30), though even this small reduction has been disputed by some researchers (31).

Although electronic records offer some benefits, they are not a long-term solution for the rapidly accelerating medical costs. Any long-term cost solution would have to focus on changing the shape of the cost curve previously shown in Figure 2.1.

Plans Touted as 'Cost-Reduction Plans' That Will Not Control Costs

Malpractice Reform

For a number of years, doctors have insisted that malpractice lawsuits are driving up the cost of medicine. Regardless of whether it is true or not, it is easy to understand why doctors would support such a view. No one enjoys being sued and doctors are no exception.

Doctors have been asking for malpractice reform. A true malpractice reform should benefit not only the doctors but also the injured patients because both sides are suffering under the present system. From the doctors' viewpoint malpractice reform primarily means some limits on their medical liability. President George W. Bush was a strong supporter of this type of malpractice reform and mentioned it often in his speeches. He assumed it was the cause of rising prices.

However, to the readers of this book, it should be clear that the true reasons for rising healthcare costs are not malpractice lawsuits but lie in the faulty markets. Any person who still thinks that limiting medical liability can have an impact on the costs, should note what happened in Texas when strict limits were placed on liability in the malpractice suits. Medical costs did not go down in Texas; rather, they increased. Chapter 9 explains why.

Medical malpractice reform is needed, though it should not be focused only on reducing malpractice awards. True malpractice reform will benefit not only the doctors but also the injured patients. Patients also need some type of automatic compensation if they are wrongfully injured by the medical system. The recommended reform is discussed in Chapter 9.

Mandating Everyone to Buy Insurance

It Does Not Solve the Long-Term Cost Problems

Under the *Affordable Care Act* (ACA), all American citizens must buy insurance or pay a penalty. This requirement of the law was the most-misunderstood and most-contested provision of the law by the political right. However, the requirement was necessary for the system to function if the insurance companies were to guarantee coverage to everyone who applied regardless of any pre-existing conditions. The reasons for this requirement are simple: if the healthy people are permitted to wait to buy insurance till they get sick, then only the sick people will buy insurance. This will raise premiums to unaffordable levels for the people in the system until the premiums rise to unsustainably high levels and the system crashes.

While the mandate to buy insurance was necessary for the successful implementation of the Affordable Care Act, it will not bring down the long-term healthcare costs as has been incorrectly argued by some. Their argument is that if we require everyone to buy insurance, then the younger, healthier population can pay for the older population and thus subsidize the costs for the elderly. In turn, when the younger people grow up and become old, they would need more healthcare but their costs, in turn, would be subsidized by new younger and healthier entrants into the market.

However there is a flaw in the above reasoning. While the law could provide more funds into the insurance pool in first year of its implementation, it will not control the long-term costs of healthcare. Here is why this strategy only lowers the costs in the year of its implementation but fails to work in subsequent years: Let us assume that the population of the United States is 300 million and that 250 million are insured with 50 million uninsured. If coverage is mandated for all, and all of the newly added individuals are perfectly healthy (a very unrealistic assumption to say the least), it would add 20 percent more funds into the coffers of insurance companies without creating any new expenses. So under this scenario the companies do not have to raise their premiums even if the healthcare rates rise by 20 percent next year.

But, what about the year after that? If the medical inflation rate is 20 percent then the second year following the implementation of the mandate, we will not have another 50 million more people to add to our pool to keep the premiums from rising again. Thus if the underlying causes of increases in medical costs are not dealt with, the strategy will not work.

Expansion of Health Savings Accounts (HSAs)

Health Savings Accounts (HSAs)[51] are already a part of our system, but some policy analysts have recommended the expansion of the concept to allow greater tax-free contributions and more flexibility on how the money can be spent from these accounts. Under current law, any person with an eligible high-deductible health plan can open up a tax-advantaged savings account to which tax-free contributions may be made and later on the money can be used for medical expenses. No tax need be paid at the time of withdrawing the money from these accounts as long as the money is spent for qualifying medical expenses.

The idea behind the health savings account is to make people more responsible for how their healthcare dollars are spent. They have a stake in how the money is used. Because it is their own money, they will be more careful in spending it, thereby putting a downward pressure on healthcare costs.

The second argument in favor of health savings accounts is that they tend to level the playing field. Because the health savings accounts are tax advantaged, the employees get some of the same tax advantages that their employers get when they buy health insurance for their employees. In this way, they tend to level the playing field between employers and employees.

The health savings accounts have met with mixed success. According to a General Accounting Office (GAO) report, most people who are reasonably healthy are satisfied with the plans and would recommend them to their friends, but they also noted that they are not for everyone.

Adding health savings accounts to the mix to solve the cost problem represents the ultimate in confused thinking. As a nation, we have been trying to put bandages on a sick healthcare system by introducing small piecemeal solutions. Health Savings Accounts are the latest such bandage. We first decided to use market mechanisms to deliver healthcare to our citizens. It was a big mistake.

Soon afterwards, we realized our mistake. Sick patients have their earning powers depleted; therefore, we realized they need some sheltering from these market forces. So, we invented the system of private health insurance to protect the sick patients against same market forces that are needed to make the free-markets work. Now, we are realizing that patients, doctors, drug companies, and hospitals are all *abusing* the system.

Instead of punishing the primary abusers, the providers, we wish to solve the problem by putting even more burden on the sick. It is like punishing the victim for the sins of the victimizer. We are implicitly assuming that it is the patients' fault that they did not put enough pressure on the providers to stop the providers from raising the prices of medicine to such dizzying heights.

The big question is can health saving accounts reduce cost? The short answer is: yes, in a limited way. They can provide some slowing down of the costs but at a psychological cost to the patient who is already sick. Even if we implement this strategy, it is too late. The price of medicine has already risen considerably for several decades because of market flaws of the past.

Our medicine has been developed under the old system. The system provided virtually unlimited amounts of money for the development of expensive medical procedures. The more expensive they were, the better it was for the providers. We allowed the providers to benefit from this system for decades. Now, we are telling the sick to be judicious while using their savings to buy this expensive medicine and help bring costs down.

Single-Payer System

In recent years the *single-payer* system has been proposed vigorously by some groups.[52] This idea is popular with many left-wing leaning individuals and groups. They see the solution as a *cure-all* for all our healthcare system ills. Yet, the proponents of the system have not explained why the solution will work or what improvements it will provide over the present system.[53]

Let us look at what this system can or cannot accomplish. And, in what shape or form is this solution likely to be implemented in the United States, if at all? In particular, we want to know if this solution will provide sustainable long-term control of healthcare costs.

First, let's clarify what we will be referring to when we use the term *single-payer*. The term *single-payer* can mean different things to different people. E.g. some only refer to the Canadian system as a single-payer system. Others like to think of the systems such as the British system *also* as a single-payer system, but these are two very different systems.

In the Canadian system, the government is the payer, but the doctors are still paid on a *fee-for-service basis* just like most of the doctors in the United States. On the other hand, in England the dominant system is the one where doctors are paid on a *salary basis*. This is a *critical* distinction.

Because of the limitations of the English language, both systems can loosely be described using the label 'single-payer,' but these systems *function* very differently. Whether doctors are paid on a fee-for-service or on a salary basis, changes the incentives for doctors. This can have a huge impact on healthcare costs. In this book, when the term *single-payer* is used, it will always refer to the Canadian-type system.

To evaluate what a single-payer system could accomplish in the United States, we can get some guidance from Medicare. Medicare is just such a system already operating in the United States for people over the age of sixty-five years. The single-payer solution could be implemented in two ways in the United States.

Implementation Strategy 1: Mandating Medicare for Everyone

Some advocates of the single-payer system have suggested moving the whole population of the United States into Medicare. If a single payer solution is adopted in the United States in the near future, it is very likely to be this type of implementation, because it would entail minimum loss to the finances of the healthcare providers[54] and possibly might mean greater income for them.

Under such a system, doctors, drug companies, and hospitals can continue to do business as usual though the providers will now have to accept payments from Medicare only. It might not be a big change for them because many of these providers are already used to being paid by Medicare. It would be a bigger loss to some health insurance companies which might now have to go out of business.[55]

It is quite easy to visualize what a single-payer solution would mean in the United States by simply looking at our Medicare system. First of all, let us examine if such a solution would control healthcare costs? A casual look at the numbers will show that Medicare is not such an efficient system after all. In 2010, Medicare spent $10,500.00 per person (2) whereas Canada spent $3,692.00 per person on healthcare (32). The higher expenditures in the United States might be partly attributed to the older U.S. population.

Canada can hold down costs because its hospitals are strictly controlled by provincial governments. Hospital costs are a major part of any medical bill, and as discussed in Chapter 1, Canadian hospitals cost only a fraction of what the American hospitals do.

Another way that Canada has kept the healthcare costs down is by limiting the *supply* of hospitals. Even though Canadian doctors, like their American counterparts, have incentives to perform more surgeries, their efforts are curbed by the limited supply of operating facilities.[56] Whereas, in the United States, the government expenses for Medicare are kept in check because recipients have to pay a 20 percent deductible for most services.Were it not for these high deductibles, Medicare costs to the government would be even higher.

If we switch to this system in America, we would probably have to require a 20 percent deductible from the insured population (just as we do from Medicare recipients), to keep government expenditures down. But the prices of medicine are already so high that *many people will still be under the threat of bankruptcy* due to this high deductible.

The total national expenditures would still not come down and they might even rise because government would have a harder time denying payments to the sick unlike what occurs with private insurers. Our hospitals are also expensive, and more numerous than in Canada, which will add to the cost.

The only advantages to the single payer system are that the claims process for patients will be much simplified (a worthwhile result in itself. [57]) and patients will have less worry about claims being denied (although there are also people who think the government will ration their healthcare).

This single-payer solution does not eliminate the major causes of the rising healthcare costs – namely *fee-for-service medicine* and the *system of insurance* to pay for this type of medicine. It was this duo that we identified in Chapter 2 as the culprit in the rising costs of healthcare. This single-payer system simply replaces the private insurance with government insurance.

Even though the single-payer solution might turn out to be better than the system that we have now (because it simplifies the claims process), it is not a long-term solution. It might even delay the real reform by side tracking the reform effort.

Implementation Strategy 2: Giving People the 'Option' of Buying into Medicare

A proposal that promises even less loss of income to the providers than the previously discussed implementation would be to allow everyone to buy into the present Medicare system *if they so choose* but not to mandate it. Giving the option does not immediately threaten the existence of the health insurance industry, although if the option proves popular, in the long run it could.

Such a system would be the same as a system with the *Public Option,* which has already been discussed in this chapter.

Likely Impact of the Affordable Care Act (Obamacare)

Strictly speaking, Obamacare is not a reform proposal, but is now the law of the land. Therefore, some readers might feel that its discussion does not belong in this chapter. However, at the time of writing this chapter, some of its provisions have not been implemented and those provisions that have been implemented are fairly recent. The full impact of the Affordable Care Act has yet to be realized. Therefore, we can speculate about the impact the law is likely to have on the future costs and the quality of healthcare.

What is Good About Obamacare?

Obamacare was enacted with a very worthy goal: to provide access to health insurance to all U.S. citizens regardless of the health or financial status of the recipients. For the first time in the history of the United States, all Americans are eligible for insurance coverage. This is particularly good news for those who had pre-existing conditions and were previously ineligible for insurance coverage. It is also good news for the poor who will now be given government subsidies to help defray the cost of insurance.

For a very long time, the United States has lagged behind other developed nations (as well as many developing nations) in providing affordable healthcare to its citizens. For these reasons, it is definitely a step in the right direction.

Another good thing about the ACA is that it takes some positive steps to control costs. For example, it attempts to monitor the system more closely to get rid of and rectify the abuses. It creates Accountable Care Organizations (ACOs) to oversee the delivery of healthcare. Other provisions deny payments to hospitals and providers when patients have to be readmitted for treatment of the same problem within a limited period after the discharge.

Shortcomings of Obamacare

Incentives in the System are Unchanged

However, despite these provisions, the law suffers from some shortcomings. The biggest shortcoming is that it keeps the *same system of provider incentives* while it tries to provide insurance to everyone.

It is an inefficient way to control costs because it tries to reduce costs by more closely *monitoring* the system rather than by *changing its incentives*. This is a much harder way of accomplishing the task because it is likely to take a lot of effort by the monitoring agencies. The providers are certain to come up with ways to bypass the efforts and game the system. The system continues to encourage more medicine and risky procedures by paying more for these. Then, it tries to monitor the abuses that result from such incentives. This is like trying to slow down an automobile by pressing both the brakes and the gas pedal at the same time.

Insurance is not the same as 'Guarantee of Care'

There are other shortcomings in the law as well. Even though Obamacare *attempts* to provide universal coverage, it essentially *fails* to do so. Having health *insurance* is not the same as a *guarantee* of care in the event of sickness. Even the subsidized insurance plans have fairly high deductibles. Many basic plans in some states come with a yearly deducible of approximately $6,500 or more. While this amount may not seem much to middle class Americans, remember that these plans are for the poor, who probably do not have this much money in their savings accounts.

Further, in case of chronic illness, this amount of money will be needed year after year. Someone, who has saved $6,500 in his or her savings account, will run out of money after the first year. Illness reduces one's ability to earn, thus the availability of insurance coverage does not necessarily mean the end of hardship for the poor, who might have to declare bankruptcy even after having insurance.

Potentially Inflationary Effect of Obamacare

Obamacare has at least one provision that can potentially *inflate medical costs.* Under the new law, insurance companies are prohibited from putting lifetime limits on benefits. While this provision is good news for those with serious and chronic diseases, whose benefits had a chance of running out in their lifetimes, this provision also provides *virtually limitless* funds into the healthcare system. This will be an *enticement* to the providers to gobble up these *unlimited* dollars.

This provision is one factor causing the rapidly rising insurance premiums that we have experienced since the enactment of the law. Insurance providers will likely respond by further increasing insurance deductibles (or raising premiums). This puts even more pressure on the sick. Thus, the law could end up *worsening the problem that it is trying to solve.*

Conclusion

Neither any of the reforms discussed above, nor Obamacare provide us with long-term solution to controlling costs. Since we have identified the cause of rising prices as the faulty market structure that results from the perverse incentives, then these incentives will have to be changed for any long term solution.

In the next chapter, we will discuss how to change these incentives in ways that will result in sustainable low-cost healthcare system. Going after the profits of health insurance industry represents only a red herring and will not bring down costs significantly nor control their long-term growth.

It is time we forget trying to tinker with the operation of insurance companies in the hope that this will significantly reduce our medical bills. Instead, let's focus on the crux of the problem: the underlying medical costs.

The health insurance industry has its problems, but trying to improve its operation to reduce underlying medical costs is like performing surgery on Peter and hoping that Paul will benefit.

CHAPTER 6

HEALTHCARE REFORM

...not everything that counts can be counted.—William Bruce Cameron

Most present day healthcare problems fall into two distinct categories. The first category contains those problems that arise from the high costs of medicine. Examples of such problems include the inability of Americans to afford medicine and patients having to declare bankruptcies because they cannot pay unreasonable and highly inflated medical bills. Many of the bankruptcies arise from the patients' inability to pay just the insurance deductibles. At the national level, high costs are straining Medicare and Medicaid programs, as well as other national resources including the resources of private American businesses.

The second category of healthcare related problems includes those issues that are related to the unsafe nature of modern medicine. Examples of these problems are the large number of deaths that routinely occur from medical mistakes and the growing number of malpractice lawsuits stemming from the practice of risky medicine.

Any reform that promises to fix the troubles in these two categories, while also promising long-term slower growth in costs is a solution we should be searching for. Ironically, it is the same features of the system that are causing both types of problems. Changing the underlying factors responsible for the rising costs can reduce the practice of unsafe medicine too.

So, let us first focus on the cost problem. In today's healthcare markets, medical procedures can run into hundreds of thousands of dollars. Lifetime costs for serious diseases such as cancer or diabetes, can reach the multi-million dollar mark. Under such a scenario, most reform proposals of the last chapter that tinker with the operation of insurance industry cannot be expected to provide significant relief from such a monumental burden of costs.

Making the insurance industry[58] more efficient might shave off a few percentage points in insurance premiums, but it will not make much of a dent in American healthcare costs that have reached dizzying heights. More importantly, it will not change the long-term pattern of growth.

No insurance company can be expected to insure its clients for a small sum of money when healthcare costs have reached such astronomical proportions. It is unreasonable to expect insurance companies to provide coverage for say $20 a month or a similar small amount when the cost of medical procedures can run into hundreds of thousands of dollars. Cancer drugs cost on average a hundred thousand dollars per year and the total costs of the disease can run into several million dollars in a lifetime.

The Crux of the Problem

Therefore, it is time we forget about trying to put slightly more efficiency in the insurance system in the hope that this will significantly reduce our medical bills. Instead, let us focus on the crux of the problem: the *underlying* medical costs.[59]

So, what is the reason for the high U.S. medical costs including high doctors' fees, or drugs that can cost hundreds of thousands of dollars per year, or hospitals that charge many times what the hospitals abroad charge?

The answer is simple. Our flawed healthcare market structure that is the result of the two pillars on which our system stands (Chapter 2). In this chapter, we may view these pillars as two legs of a monster of a system that is creating the uncontrollable price spiral.

The Two-Legged Monster

The two pillars on which our system stands might be a blessing for doctors and other healthcare providers, because of the wealth it generates for them, but the system is a curse for the rest of the society. For most Americans, the system not only burdens them with the costs, but by encouraging the over-use of unsafe medicine, opens the gates for medical errors and the ensuing medical injuries. This monster must be slain in order for us to arrive at a safer, cheaper, sustainable system that promises moderate (perhaps negative) rate of growth in costs.

As a reminder from Chapter 2, here are the two legs of this monster:

1. Fee-for-service payments to doctors regardless of the results. In addition, the practice of making higher payments for more risky medicine.

2. Payments for these services through third-party insurance companies.

It is easy to see how the first leg of the monster contributes to the use of too much medicine as well as unsafe medicine while the second leg contributes to higher prices because patients are now not responsible for the costs. Doctors and other providers can put their hands in the pockets of insurance companies, that are loaded with money.

The reader should also note that the first provision is the result of attempting to deliver a product such as healthcare, through *market mechanisms*. Since health is not easily quantifiable (a product should be quantifiable if markets are to be effectively used for its delivery), we decided to pay doctors on a fee-for-service basis without regard to any benefit that their services might provide. This was the first mistake.

Since sickness creates financial need and takes away a person's ability to earn, we introduced insurance to pay for these services still insisting that markets must be used for healthcare delivery. This was the second mistake.

Both these provisions favor doctors and providers at the expense of patients. That is why the current system is a panacea for the providers but a bane for consumers. Cut off either of the legs of this monster and you have a more manageable system. For example, if we cut off its second leg by start requiring that everyone must pay for medicine out of his or her own savings (rather than relying on insurance), prices of medicine will come tumbling down.

This will change medicine as we know it. Few doctors will insist that patients get open heart surgeries. Highly effective aspirin and garlic will be in more demand. The deaths and complications that result from unsafe surgeries will go to almost zero. The resulting malpractice lawsuits also will be greatly diminished.

There will be very few hip replacement surgeries. There will be very few back-surgeries or any other surgeries for that matter.

Cancer drugs currently can cost around $100,000 per year or more. Many cancer patients are elderly and unable to work. So, under the system just mentioned, it will be impossible for drug companies to ask for these amounts from their patients. They will have to sell their drugs at cheaper prices or not at all. Or, drug companies might have to come up with cheaper drugs that patients might be able to afford.Therefore, people would have to rely more on inexpensive herbs or food to manage their illness (Medicating with herbs can be very effective though very few people try it.)

Now, let us consider what type of a system we would end up with if we could cut off the first leg of the monster. This would mean that we pay doctors only in proportion to the health benefit their services deliver. Unfortunately, as we have already established, it is not possible to quantify health so such a system is hard to conceive; so we will not consider this type of a solution further.

Why Are We Still Struggling to Come Up with a Satisfactory System?

The necessity of quantifying health occurs only if we try to use markets to deliver healthcare to our citizens. If we are willing to open ourselves to the possibility of delivering care through non-market mechanisms, we need not be able to quantify health.

At the bottom of our inability to find a satisfactory system lies our reluctance to abandon markets as a mechanism for delivery of an unquantifiable product such as healthcare. While markets have worked beautifully in many areas of the economy and are the preferred way to produce national wealth, they have not functioned well for the delivery of health for reasons just mentioned and for other reasons noted in Chapter 2.

Our present healthcare payment system avoided the measurement of health by paying doctors for procedures regardless of their benefit. But, this has not worked well.

In the United States, the doctor who performs the procedure is usually the *same* doctor who recommended it. So, he or she has an incentive to recommend the most expensive procedure he or she knows how to perform. The most expensive procedures are also the riskiest. Even if the procedure kills the patient, the doctor will get paid. This form of a payment system is neither good at controlling costs nor is good for the patients' health.

In fact, fee-for-service is not a good idea for many type of businesses. It is especially troublesome in those areas of the economy that employ advanced technologies and specialized knowledge because there is a big informational gap between the consumer and the provider. In medicine the term fee-for-service has taken on entirely new meaning: payments without regards to results.

For example, it is not a good idea even in businesses such as auto repair where it is the mechanic who is in a position to first diagnose the problem, then perform the repair, and then charge according to the procedure performed. But, in auto repair, the situation is less serious. Usually the owner of the automobile is healthy enough to bargain or to go to another shop for comparison. The results of the repair are also more easily apparent and the consumers are more demanding because they are paying for the repair from their own pocket.

In healthcare, the sickness of the patient generally prevents comparison shopping. There is also a large information gap between the patient and the doctor. Most people are not able to accurately evaluate if it was the medicine that helped them or if their condition improved because of their body's healing powers or if it was because of a placebo effect.

It is not known if we will ever be able to accurately quantify health and be able to pay healthcare professionals accordingly. Meanwhile, the need to reform our system has become more critical. We must do something now before the system wrecks the economy while continuing to harm or kill patients.

How to Eliminate Perverse Incentives in the Present System

The good news is that just because we do not know how to quantify health does not mean that there are no other ways of paying the healthcare providers. One option is to pay doctors on a *salary-only* basis.

In fact, in the absence of any other way to quantify health, paying doctors on a salaried basis seems to be our only satisfactory option. It is not a perfect solution. Paying doctors on salaried basis is a mixed blessing. Even though it removes incentives for doctors to dispense unnecessary and unsafe medicine, it does not directly offer any *additional* financial rewards (other than the salary) for healing patients. In this system, the additional rewards to physicians must be of a psychological nature and must come from the satisfaction one gets from healing the sick.

However, it is far better to provide no extra financial incentives beyond salary than to provide the wrong ones. We only want those people in the medical profession who are genuinely interested in healing others, rather than those who are attracted to it for the money.

We will see later in this chapter how implementation of a system that involves salaried doctors can reduce the costs of healthcare system to achieve these objectives. For now, let us examine some healthcare delivery systems that pay doctors exclusively on salary and are operational in the United States or abroad. Perhaps these systems can give us a hint as to what kind of a system would be best for us.

Current Systems in the United States and Abroad Where Doctors are Salaried

Salaried Systems Provide Guidance for Change

Many hospitals in the United States employ some of their doctors on a salary basis. Some Health Maintenance Organizations (HMOs), such as Kaiser Permanente, also employ their doctors on a salary basis

Other organizations in the United States that employ doctors on salaried basis are organizations such as Cleveland Clinic in Ohio and the Mayo Clinic in Minnesota. These institutions provide excellent services. They have been praised for their efficiency by experts in the field (33) and have even been suggested as models to be emulated. President Obama praised them and said that these can serve as models for reform in the United States. Many Canadians who come to the United States for surgeries often make use of these institutions.

The British system

The model that should interest us is being practiced outside the country: the British System.

Adopting the British system (or a modification of it) can save us a ton of money in healthcare costs and enable us to provide free healthcare to all Americans without imposing any new taxes. Later, it will be explained how this is possible. But first let us examine more fully what British system is and how it works.

In the context of this book, when the term British system is used, it would mean the system being used in the United Kingdom. That is, in its four constituent countries: England, Scotland, Wales and Northern Ireland. Though all four systems are run by a separate authority, they are so similar in their structure and operation, that for the purposes of this book, we will treat them as a single system. Together, they will be labeled as the British system.

Even though most Americans like to think of the British system as an all government-run socialist system, it is not an accurate description of the system. Actually U.K. has two systems running in parallel.

People in U.K. are allowed to buy private health insurance just like in the United States and use fee-for-service medicine if they so desire.

However, the dominant system, used by over 90 percent of the British, is the free-system run by their National Health Service (NHS). Understanding the operation of this system is critical because it is used by the vast majority of the population, and therefore determines the cost of medicine in England.

The keys to the low costs produced by the British system are in its two main features. First and most important: all the doctors in its National Healthcare Service are paid a salary. Second, the hospitals in the system are government-owned.

On the other hand, the high costs of healthcare for most of the U.S. population are determined by its healthcare system that 1. Pays doctors on a fee-for service basis, through private insurance. 2. The hospitals are privately owned and operated.

The doctors who work for the NHS can moonlight and provide additional services on fee-for-service basis if they so choose. There are very few doctors in the U.K. who earn all their income entirely through private practice.

The attraction of the British system lies in the fact that it eliminates the perverse doctor incentives, making it cheap. But because it is also totally free, it effectively controls the costs even for those who want to use fee-for-service system. The costs in fee-for-service system can never go up very much because people always have the option of giving up their fee-for-service medicine and relying on the free system. It all works because the free-system is good enough so that people can rely on it and don't mind giving up fee-for-service medicine.

Observing the British system can give us clues to cost savings if we were to duplicate the British system in America. We can accurately gauge the costs as well as any potential problems we might have simply by observing their system. It is a great system but it can be improved. So, if we were to adopt this system, it would make sense to make further improvements to it after adopting it.

Will duplication of this system in our country alter the incentives of healthcare providers enough to reduce the healthcare costs sufficiently for us? How much can we expect to save if we make this change? These are the questions we must answer.

Estimated Cost Savings by Adopting the British System

Let us assume that we switch to the British system. Vast majority of doctors will now work in government-owned facilities. All hospitals will be government-owned. The question we would like to answer is: how much effect will this have on the costs of healthcare in America?

It is not difficult to estimate how much we can save simply by making this change. Using this system to deliver medicine, Great Britain provides healthcare at 40 percent of the cost (per person) of that of the United States (34). By simply switching to this system, America could immediately cut its costs to 40 percent of the levels of current healthcare costs.

Let us briefly examine what kind of impact this can have on our national budget. In 2014, we spent about $3.03 trillion[60] on healthcare (including all private and government spending). Out of this total sum, about $1.23 trillion were spent by the U.S. government on Medicare, Medicaid, CHIP, V.A.,and the Department of Defense (2).

Even if we decided to implement the British System in the United States without any other improvements, it could bring the medical costs in America to about 40 percent of what they are now.

Assuming 2014 figures, this change will bring down the total U.S. healthcare expenditure to about 1.23 trillion dollars. This is the same amount the U.S. government spent on all its healthcare programs. This means that the U.S. government can pay this entire bill for all the U.S. citizens with what it is currently spending. without imposing any new taxes.

In other words, a change in our system of delivery of medicine can also relieve one *major worry* for our citizens: the worry about their health. No one need buy health insurance. No one need worry about going bankrupt if sickness strikes. No one need lose his or her lifetime earnings at the end of one's life.

In addition, by changing the system, we will also change the shape of the cost curve shown in Chapter 2 because we will remove the fundamental drivers of cost that were responsible for the hockey stick shape. Since Americans would not be paying monthly insurance premiums, they would not feel the compulsion to get something back for their money. Doctors would not recommend unnecessary expensive surgeries since they would have nothing to gain financially by such recommendations.

Benefits of Switching to the British System

What are some of the obvious advantages this system will have, not only for the individual citizens but also for the nation as a whole?

Benefits for Patients

A Dream System for U.S. Citizens.[61]

For starters, the proposed system will provide free care for all U.S. citizens regardless of their income or assets. No one would be required to buy health insurance. No money would be needed to pay for coinsurance, deductibles, or many of the prescription medications. Wherever necessary, the transportation to the hospital could also be provided free in medical emergencies.

The energy of our citizens could then be used for more productive pursuits because guaranteed coverage would also mean the end of worry about having to declare bankruptcy because of medical bills or having to die destitute because of end-of-life medical costs.

Benefits for Private Industry

Since the government would now provide free healthcare to all citizens, there would be no need for private companies to provide health insurance to their employees. This would reduce manufacturing costs for American products, making America once again more competitive in the world. One reason for recent bankruptcies of General Motors and Chrysler Corporation was that healthcare costs were adding a significant burden to their manufacturing costs. Our American healthcare system is a cancer that threatens to grow and consume the healthy sectors of our economy. This would be great way to stop this cancer cold in its tracks.

Benefits for the Government

One of the reasons the Social Security system could run into financial problems in the future is because of rising Medicare costs. If the future healthcare costs keep on rising at the pace at which they are, it would be almost impossible to maintain a system that will keep on paying the retirees. A great way to keep Social Security and Medicare solvent in the future is to change our healthcare system.

Too Good to be True?

Thus far, we focused on the comparison with the British System to show how costs can be reduced in our own system. Although this is easily shown by direct comparison with the British System, some of us might still be skeptical about how it is possible to achieve that and whether we will have to make sacrifices in terms of quality or convenience if we adopt such a system.

But such sacrifices will not be required. There are common misunderstandings that make it hard to accept the possibility of achieving such spectacular results without major sacrifices by Americans. Two misconceptions keep us from understanding how a system can provide free coverage without the need to impose new taxes.

1. First, many Americans believe that the present-day prices of medicine in the United States are fair prices and would not change if we had a different system. They believe if medicine is to be made available for free to everyone, it must be at the current prices; therefore, universal free coverage will raise their taxes.

Most people fail to see that the prices are a function of the system that is being used to provide the delivery of medicine. As discussed in Chapter 2, our healthcare system is not a free market system at all. In the present system, payments are being made by a third party only for procedures and not for healing. This has highly inflated the prices of medicine.

2. Second, many believe that modern medicine, based predominantly on drugs and surgeries, is "scientific" and will not change if we change our system. (We will revisit this topic again in Chapter 8.) The belief that medicine is a science is rooted in the observation that since it is being recommended by a scientifically trained doctor, this means that medicine must also be a "science."

Many people believe that since there can be only one scientific truth, therefore the treatment recommended by their doctor must be the *only* effective way to treat their illness. But they are wrong. It is just an *opinion* of the doctor. Consultation with another doctor might yield different advice.

The prices of medicine can also be brought down by choosing safer and cheaper herbal medications instead of unsafe medicines based on drugs and surgeries. Contrary to the popular belief, many herbal medications that are safer can also be very effective as we will discuss in Chapter 8.

The readers should also note that many of the surgical procedures routinely performed by doctors are *not evidence based*. The effectiveness of most surgical procedures has not been adequately studied. It is extremely difficult to directly evaluate the effectiveness of the surgical procedures because it would be impossible to carry out double-blind studies (such as those used in drug research) to evaluate surgical effectiveness.

The standard double-blind studies (used to evaluate drugs)[62] would require performing fake surgeries on some patients, which poses ethical problems. The effectiveness of the surgeries must therefore be evaluated indirectly or not at all. The effectiveness of many surgeries, even the most expensive of all surgeries, such as heart surgeries has been vigorously debated even within the medical community.

The current practice of medicine uses mostly those procedures and surgeries that are very expensive. These expensive procedures are the very procedures that are also unsafe. But, the fee to perform these unsafe and risky procedures and surgeries is higher since they are perceived to require more skill. Thus, the result of our incentive system is that we have very unsafe medicine being practiced at very high prices. Once we change the incentives, we will also change the types of surgeries that will be performed, and there will be fewer of these. In time, more research can be done to develop more of the cheaper and safer methods of healing; although the problem is not the lack of information about safe healing methods. The bigger problem is that these are being ignored under our current system of incentives.

Some Common Objections to Switching to a Mostly Government System

No matter how advantageous the British system can be for the United States, some individuals would object to adopting a government system for healthcare delivery. In the following paragraphs, we will discuss various objections that are likely to be put forward against switching to this system.

These are likely to be fears about waiting in lines, lack of choice, and rationing that might occur in a government-based system. Some people might also worry that if it is not a fee-for-service system, the doctors will not be as motivated to help the patients. Others might worry that such a system would not produce new research for new diseases and doctors in such a system would not experiment with new ways to treat the diseases.

First, however, let us be clear that just because a free government system is being proposed, this *does not mean the abolition of the private system altogether.* In addition to the system that we already have, we should adopt a parallel high quality government system that covers everyone and the doctors in this free system should be salaried.

The proposed additional system, therefore, will give *more* choice to everyone, not *less.* Both systems can run in parallel and later in the section, we will see why the combined cost of the two systems will be less than the cost of single system that we have now. The free system will also bring down the cost of the private system because there will be less need to use the private system.

The better the free system the less demand there would be for the private system; therefore, the cheaper the private system would be. Thus, the proposed change will not just benefit those taxpayers who choose to use the free system, but also extend to those who would like to use the private system.

Those who do not wish to take advantage of the free system will not have to do so. Introduction of a free system will not impinge on anyone's freedom to use the private system. Those who like our present system, can continue with it and never have to bother with the free government system. However, providing a parallel free system will reduce the cost of the private system because people now have a choice of using the free system.

England has a two-tier system like this. Since such a system reduces costs by changing the doctors' incentives, it only costs about 40 percent (per person) of the cost of the U.S. system. In other words, having two systems, one of which is totally free but covered by salaried doctors, can bring down *the combined cost of two systems to less than what the government is spending now on healthcare.*[63]

Long Lines for Surgeries

One of the biggest fears that people have is that if we switch to a British-like system, then they might have to wait for needed surgeries. This fear comes mainly from the fact that many Canadians come here for surgeries because they do not want to wait in line in Canada.

Therefore, let's be clear that the system being recommended in this book is *not* the Canadian system. We need not worry about the shortcomings of the Canadian system. The British do not routinely come to the United States for surgeries. It would be unwise, because the costs in the U.S. are very high but in Britain they are available for free if people are only willing to wait for non-emergency surgeries.

For emergency surgeries, there is no wait even in England. If British citizens buy inexpensive (compared to U.S. prices) supplemental insurance, they do not have to wait *even* for non-emergency surgeries.

Why do Lines Occur?[64]

In general, lines occur in those markets where a product is available below the free-market price. A lower price than that determined by the laws of supply and demand generates greater demand. Demand at a lower than market price can exceed the available supply, thus creating lines or waiting periods. For example, if the U.S. government were to use price controls on gas prices, and force the gas to be sold at below-market prices, you will see lines at gas stations.

In any country where medicine is totally free, the cost to patients is essentially zero (at the point of delivery). Therefore, the demand for medicine will be greater than if people had to pay. So, you can have lines if medicine is free (unless we lower the demand by informing people about the risks of medicine). The situation is not really that bad as long as you can avoid lines by paying for the medicine either directly out of your own pocket or through insurance. In fact, the availability of a free product can actually bring down the price of the product for those who want to pay for it.

In any society where people understand the risks associated with surgeries, the demand for them would be low and the lines would be shorter.

Doctors minimize the risks of medicine due to the profit motive. These providers are in a position to shape public opinion, to convince consumers that medical procedures are less risky and more desirable than they really are. This creates more demand for medicine in countries where the medicine is practiced for profit.

Why do Canadians Come to the United States for Surgeries?

The major reason Canadians come to the United States for non-emergency surgeries is because of provisions in the Canadian healthcare laws that prohibit Canadians from going to a private doctor in Canada if the disease is covered by the Canadian healthcare system. These provisions in Canadian laws have been *purposely added by the legislatures to make the system egalitarian* and prohibit the rich from gaining an advantage over those less fortunate.

A Canadian system is not being recommended here,[65] but even if we were (in a hypothetical case) to adopt a Canadian-type system, it would be up to us to add laws to make our system as egalitarian as Canada's.

Choice

Many people believe they will always have less choice in any government system. There could be two different types of choices that individuals might be worried about: the choice in selecting a doctor and the choice of getting pertinent treatments.

As far as choosing a doctor, the same amount of choice can be provided under the new system as insurance companies now provide. There is absolutely no reason why the same number of choices will not be available under a system that pays doctors on a salary basis rather than a system that pays the doctors on a fee-for-service basis. Even in our current system, some entities such as the HMOs, where doctors are paid on salary, give you the choice of a doctor. In England too patients can choose their physician.

Another type of choice is *the choice of procedures* that a patient might want. This is the aspect of choice that people fear losing the most. Under the present system, most patients undergo treatments recommended by their doctors. They might think they are choosing the best treatment for themselves, but they are heavily influenced by their doctors.

If people knew what is best for them, they would not even need a doctor's recommendation. Implicit in the visit to your doctor is your admission that you do not know what is best for you. Under the current system, the procedures that are recommended are those which are also in the *interest of the doctor* rather than the patient *alone*. Although patients might feel *good* that the procedure they are getting is the most *expensive* one, the most expensive procedures are also the *riskiest*. The expensive procedures benefit the providers while subjecting the patients to risk.

Under these circumstances it might be best for the patients to put their trust in the government-run system. A salaried doctor will recommend a procedure based on patient's needs alone because the doctor has no profit motive.

The present system also limits choice whether patients realize it or not. In the current system, private insurance companies routinely deny care that the patients ask for. What is more egregious is that this denial often occurs because of the profit motive of the private insurance companies.

Rationing

The private insurance companies have been rationing our healthcare for years whether we are aware of it or not. Before the passage of the Affordable Care Act, all healthcare policies had lifetime limits. Once the lifetime limit was exhausted, people were on their own. Yes, it was rationed care.

In addition, the insurance companies could deny coverage for pre-existing conditions. After the initial coverage with one policy was exhausted, it was nearly impossible to get coverage from another company. So, the system posed a risk for everyone in the system.

If you have a chronic or other serious medical condition, with today's prices, the lifetime limits of private insurance can be exhausted rather quickly. The prices of expensive surgeries can run into hundreds of thousands of dollars. If there is a complication, and you have to be re-admitted to the hospital, all your limits could easily be exhausted in one medical event.

Even though some people were against the passage of Obamacare because they thought it might ration their healthcare, the opposite has happened. The ACA prohibits lifetime limits on insurance policies. Therefore, a big risk has been eliminated (Although the inflationary effects of this provision remain to be seen: the rapid rise in premiums since the passage of the law can be partly attributed to this provision).

Only time will tell how long this type of un-rationed expenditures on healthcare can continue without adverse market effects, but note that the desire to have un-rationed care is an irrational one, because everything that we want in this world is rationed by the money we have. For example if you were required to pay for medicine with your own money (not the insurance company's money), you would only be able to buy so much medicine until your money ran out.

Under such a system, if you were poor, you might not be able to afford surgeries that you thought you needed. Even in the present system, when we buy health insurance, we are trying to ration our monthly payments to a limited amount in the hope that we might be able to draw upon greater reserves of the insurance company should sickness strike.

But, if anyone thinks that a system can be devised in which all participants can limit their own contribution but be able to withdraw unlimited amounts of money from the same money pool, they are hoping for an unrealizable dream. The government systems as well as private insurance systems work because most participants are healthy and others are reasonable with their demands and do not expect unlimited un-rationed services.

Under the system proposed in this chapter, necessary and reasonable care can be provided to all because costs will not change significantly with the type of care.

Incentives for Doctors

Some people worry that if doctors are paid on a salary basis, then they would lose the incentive to work hard on behalf of patients to make them well. But, we must keep in mind that *in the current system there are no incentives to make patients healthy. Current incentives to doctors are for performing procedures.*

It is far better not to give extra financial incentives to make people well than to give wrong incentives that encourage more procedures to be performed on patients that subject them to unnecessary risk.

Another tool that we have these days but was not available to us some years ago is the internet. Patients can always post their evaluations about their experiences with a doctor on the internet and thus provide feedback about the doctor's performance. This feedback can work as a valuable motive for doctors to work hard.[66]

Any supplemental research needed to assist medical practitioners or to improve medical treatments can be done separately at a government facility, such as the National Institutes of Health (NIH) or at universities–just as it is being done now.

Why Recommend Two Parallel Systems Instead of Just One System?

Earlier in the book, we mentioned that the way to solve the problem of healthcare costs was to abolish all fee-for-service payments to the doctors. Yet, a two-tier approach is being recommended here that does not eliminate fee-for-service altogether. This does not negate the earlier recommendations made in this book, but the recommendation of a two-tier system does need some justification.

The two tier system is not the most efficient solution for controlling prices. The most efficient way to control costs would be to allow only one free national system run by salaried doctors and to prohibit the availability of fee-for-service medicine altogether.

However, under such a scenario, any U.S citizen wanting a surgery or a medical procedure not available under the free system would either have to forgo such a procedure or go outside the country to get it. It would not matter if one were a billionaire or very poor; all would have to either do without certain medical procedures or travel to another country to get them. While this would be an extreme form of an egalitarian system and the best approach for controlling costs, such a system would be too restrictive and, therefore, unacceptable to most Americans, who are accustomed to having their freedoms. So, we are not recommending this solution.

The second most effective solution for controlling costs would be to have a free national system but allow the availability of fee-for-service medicine *only to those* who can afford to pay the *entire* cost for medical procedures out of pocket. Anyone who does not have enough money to buy this type of medicine with out-of-pocket money (in other words,without the help of insurance) would be forced to use the free system or forgo the procedure.

Under such a scenario, the costs of fee-for-service medicine will fall drastically, because of the availability of totally free medicine for all. Everyone will have access to the free system if they so choose, though they might have to wait their turn for some treatments.

The second solution, like the previous one, might not be acceptable to many Americans in the early stages of reform. It might be too drastic a change for most people to adopt in the short run, but we must consider this type of system in the *long run*.

The suggested two-tier system would satisfy most Americans, even though it does not as effectively control the costs as the previous two solutions. How much cost reduction can we expect if we adopt a two tiered system? The question is not hard to answer, because the British system offers a *working model* as an example. Even though the British allow two systems to run in parallel, they are still able to provide healthcare at 40 percent of the cost per person of that in the United States

The reason the two-tiered system in Britain is able to cut costs is because the *dominant system* in England is the *free* system. Very few people *need* to buy supplementary insurance as an *absolute necessity*. As soon as the prices charged by the providers in the fee-for-service system tend to rise, people have the option of ditching their supplemental insurance and relying totally on the free system. In other words, the *free public system is good enough so that people can do without buying supplemental insurance.*

If we want to save money on national healthcare expenditures by introducing a free-system, we will also have to make the free system *good enough* so that it becomes the *dominant* system that most people *want* to use. If the free system is not good enough for the the majority of Americans, the cost reductions would not be adequate.

Conclusion

Any effective control of costs of medicine must be based on *changing the incentives involved in the delivery of medicine.* The fee-for-service system for paying doctors must be changed if doctors' incentives are to be changed. In absence of any good way of measuring or quantifying health, the salaried system seems to be our only option. The cost-benefits of salaried system can be estimated by observing the already functioning British system, which covers its citizens at 40 percent of the cost (per person) of what it costs in the United States.

Since the U.S government already spends a significant amount of money on healthcare, changing the system to a British-like system will save the federal government enough money to provide free health coverage to all citizens while spending same money that it does currently.[67] This change can be made without forcing anyone to use the new system, but by giving the people the *option* to buy private insurance if they do not want to use the free system.

Even for those who wish to buy private insurance, the system would end up costing less than what they are spending now on insurance premiums plus taxes.

Can the proposed new system be implemented in the current political environment? This topic will be considered next.

Change to the new system need not be accomplished in a single step. It can be a gradual process. Since people over the age of sixty-five are currently covered by Medicare, and the government is already responsible for paying for a major part of their healthcare expenses, changes in these programs should take priority.

CHAPTER 7

OVERCOMING POLITICAL DIFFICULTIES IN CHANGING THE SYSTEM AND THE FUTURE OF HEALTHCARE

Gradual Steps to Ultimate Change

"A good idea is about 10 percent and implementation and hard work, and luck is 90 percent." - Guy Kawasaki

In the previous chapter, we examined the changes that we can make to our system to bring down the costs of healthcare. However, no one should be under the illusion that it will be politically easy to make changes in the current healthcare system. The present system has been in place for several decades, and it has benefited the healthcare industry at the expense of society, which has had to bear its costs while it has generated a tremendous amount of wealth for the healthcare providers. Through political lobbying and subtle influencing of public opinion, providers have resisted any attempts to make fundamental changes in the way medicine is paid for.

The past illustrates how difficult it is to change healthcare in the United States. Since the time of President Harry Truman, many presidents have attempted to make changes to the system; yet, changes have been slow to come. At every step, these changes were opposed by the special interests, and these groups have been successful in convincing the most vulnerable in our society that a free system of medicine is actually bad for them, simply because it can be labelled as socialized medicine.

Similarly, they have convinced the more well-to-do Americans that more medicine is a good thing even though the providers know full well that all modern medicine has a potential to do harm. The prices of medicine have reached the point where the rich and poor alike are at risk.

However, as the price of medicine continues to skyrocket upwards, more and more people are becoming skeptical of the present system. The tide of public opinion, as well as political opinion, has slowly been shifting in favor of changing the system. After years of unsuccessful attempts to bring major changes to the system, the recent successful passage of the Patient Protection and Affordable Care Act is a testament to the changing attitudes of the public as well as politicians.

For the first time in U.S. history, those wanting a change actually staged demonstrations on the streets to show their support for changing the system. They expressed support for President Obama's bill. These demonstrations were in opposition to the opponents of change, who in the past had been the more vocal group. The bill eventually passed, albeit by the narrowest of margins.

This rising tide of changing public opinion, the growing national budget problems, the bleak picture of the future of Social Security (due to rising medical costs), the rising burden of healthcare costs on private industry–all these factors combined–can generate enough political impetus and create an opportunity for making fundamental changes to the system.

In addition, the ACA *actually puts more financial burden on the government* because it has to *provide subsidies to the poor.* This will make the budget situation more acute. Making changes to the system, as suggested in the last chapter, might be the only way to sustain a viable healthcare system over the long run.

Therefore, the rest of the chapter offers some suggestions on how we can make these changes in this tough political environment.

Implementing the British System in America

As was previously mentioned, duplicating the British system in America can cut our healthcare costs to 40 percent of the present costs. Now, we will examine what efforts would be required for the massive switch-over to this system.

Such a switch would necessitate that every city in the United States would have at least one hospital and possibly several more clinics open to all American citizens and staffed with *doctors employed on a salaried basis.* These facilities would look somewhat like Kaiser Permanente healthcare centers that Kaiser Permanente maintains in several big cities in the country. *No one visiting these centers would need to prove eligibility based on financial status* because the healthcare would be provided free to everyone who visits the facility. Only thing one might have to prove is U.S. citizenship or permanent residency.

At first, the building of new facilities might seem like a monumental task. Yet, let us not forget that during the years1946-1974, the U.S. government completed a similar project under the auspices of the Hill-Burton Act. The program was responsible for the construction of hospitals in many of the under-served areas of the country. A significant number of the hospitals all over the United States operating today were built under this program.

Medicare and Medicaid Programs Should be the First Programs Slated for Change

Changing to the new system need not be accomplished in a single step. It can be a gradual process. Since people over the age of sixty-five are currently covered by Medicare, and the federal government is already responsible for paying for a major part of their healthcare expenses, changes in these programs should take priority.

Because of its spending power, government can easily implement changes in the delivery of healthcare to the program recipients, if the recipients also support these changes. To get support from the recipients of Medicare, all the government has to do is to *ease the financial burden on these recipients while reducing its own expenditures*.

Presently, even after getting coverage through Medicare, our seniors are stuck with payments for deductibles and co-pays, which can be a substantial burden for seniors with limited resources.

Therefore, our seniors would welcome an easing of their burden. The government would also save money because delivering medicine through salaried doctors is considerably cheaper than using the fee-for-service approach.

However, a complete change into a new system even at the Medicare level need not be implemented overnight. The program outlined in the last chapter requires delivery of medicine through government-owned facilities *staffed with salaried doctors*. This means that the government will have to spend time and money to build these facilities. Alternatively, it can take over already existing city or county hospitals—many of which are now operating at a loss. These facilities would then have to be staffed by doctors paid solely by salaries.

Large Cities Could be the Best Places to Start Implementation

Although the Medicare and Medicaid recipients are spread all over the country, a significant number live in or around large cities. These population centers offer the best opportunity to start the implementation of the system. In these cities, the transportation problems for the elderly to reach the healthcare facilities would be minimal compared to the problems faced by seniors in rural areas.

The large metro areas also offer another advantage. Many hospitals in these cities are operating at a loss. These are supported with financial help of city, county, or state governments. Having the federal government take over the hospitals to provide healthcare to the elderly and the indigent should be a welcome relief for these governments. The federal government will also benefit from the takeover, because it could save on the money it is now spending to pay for the same services using the far more costly *fee-for-service* method.

To kick-start the change, Medicare can offer totally free healthcare to those recipients who live in these areas and choose to use this new system. These recipients can also be offered free transportation to the hospital. The seniors who refuse to accept free-care under the new system but want to opt for the fee-for-service type of medicine should have their deductibles raised significantly to discourage their use of such medicine. Most likely, most elderly and poor will welcome the totally free system.

Subsequent Expansion of the Program

The delivery of healthcare to Medicare patients can represent the first step in the gradual changeover to the British type of system for everyone in the country. The next logical step would be to bring people into the system who are covered under Medicaid plus those who will be getting subsidies under the newly enacted Patient Protection and Affordable Care Act.

Just as in the case of Medicare patients, these people should also welcome the free medicine in place of a system that at present requires them to pay coinsurance and co-pays even after receiving the subsidies. Considering the high prices of healthcare, the coinsurance payments can be a burden on many individuals and families. We must not forget that although the Affordable Care Act will subsidize premiums, coinsurance costs would still have to be borne by the insured.

Even after people get health insurance through Patient Protection and Affordable Care Act, our healthcare system will remain a scary domain for most Americans. The yearly out-of-pocket costs in many government-subsidized plans can be as high as $6500 or more. This is a significant burden for low income people, many of whom could still be forced into bankruptcy (35).

Once the system is in place for Medicare, Medicaid, and recipients of subsidies, it can then be opened to the general public.

Offering Doctors Free or Subsidized Education

One potential problem might be the staffing of the government healthcare facilities with salaried doctors. Doctors might have some reluctance to accept salaried-only positions because of various reasons. For example, some new medical graduates could still be paying for the student loans they took out to finance their medical education.[68]

To encourage these doctors to work on a salary basis, it might be a good idea to forgive their student loans in return for their willingness to accept employment at the government owned hospitals and facilities. Working on salaried basis can offer some advantages for the doctors, too. For example, they do not have to worry about defending themselves against malpractice lawsuits. This responsibility will be borne by their employer. A similar strategy is already being used by VA department, which pays for the medical education of doctors in return for theircommitment to work in the VA facilities for a certain number of years.[69]

Possible Further Improvements

Once we have implemented the system to cover everyone in the country in the way previously discussed, our national healthcare costs will come down significantly. Assuming our system is about as efficient as the British system, our national costs in a few years should be reduced to 40 percent of what they are now, enabling full coverage to everyone without having to impose new taxes. *We will also have removed the fundamental causes that are responsible for the cost-curve of Figure 2.1, by changing the system* of delivery of medicine. This means that we do not have to worry about future healthcare costs rising at rates that are many times the rate of general inflation.

And, since the Medicare costs affect the expenditures on Social Security, this will help in controlling and securing the future of Social Security and keeping it solvent.

Can We Make Our System Cheaper and Better than the British System?

Even after we have made these changes to our system, we need not stop here. We can go much further in enacting laws that will develop a better system at costs less than they are in Britain.

To put our country on such a path, we would need to ponder a few more questions. One such issue is drug patents. We must consider whether we should abolish awarding patents for developing new drugs.

Drug Patents

The primary reasons for the ubiquitous use of drugs in modern medicine were discussed in Chapter 3. As we mentioned , drugs serve the needs of the doctors more than the needs of the patients. Also, as discussed earlier, doctors are financially rewarded for seeing as many patients as possible in a short period of time. Their income is based on how many patients they see rather than how much time they spend or the quality of the time they spend with each patient. Writing prescription provides a quick and easy way to see more patients in a short time.

By changing the method of payment to doctors, we also reduce the need for drugs. When doctors are paid a salary, they can spend more time with patients without fearing the loss of business. They will then have the time to provide advice on healing methods, nutritious food, herbs, and lifestyle changes without risking loss of income or without the fear of losing the patient.

However, in the near future, there could be some role for drugs in healing, though at a reduced level. The question before us is whether we should continue to award drug patents for the few drugs that we might still need.

Awarding patents to private companies is not the only way to develop drugs. When we award patents, we limit research to only those drugs and substances that have a profit potential for the patent holder. These substances are a small subset of the total number of substances found in nature that have the potential to heal. In other words, the practice of granting patents will only lead us to those substances for which patents can be awarded. These substances are necessarily very expensive and usually have harmful side effects.

The other way is to use public money for drug research and research into natural substances that have potential healing powers. Currently, a lot of the fundamental research into diseases and their treatments is being done at the the National Institutes of Health (NIH) and in Universities with funding from NIH. Such efforts funded by public money can be strengthened for finding newer drugs as well as non-drug treatments.

This would be a better way to accomplish our goals, because now research can also include the use of plants and herbs for healing. Many drugs currently being used have been derived from plants. Use of these plants in their natural form can offer the same benefits while being cheaper and safer.

A lot of research on the healing properties of substances found in nature *already exists*. Many excellent research papers have been published by universities throughout the world and can be easily retrieved by going to websites such as *www.pubmed.gov*. Yet, doctors are ignoring this research. The changed system of incentives for doctors will encourage doctors to make greater use of this knowledge.

One of the big advantages of using natural substances (that have been consumed by humans for centuries) for treatment of diseases is that we need not run expensive human trials to evaluate the safety of these substances. *Safety is a big issue only with human-made patented drugs* that our bodies are not used to handling. Patented drugs appear as unrecognized substances in the human body and can have large number of harmful side effects. Therefore, the drug companies must carry out extensive safety trials. Trials are expensive and sometimes harm the unwitting human volunteers who are willing to be used as guinea pigs. Natural substances would require fewer such trials and do less all round harm in the process.

Conclusion

The system can be changed in relatively painless ways by making incremental changes. Changes should be implemented first in the Medicare system and then expanded to cover the rest of the population. Abolishing the patent system for drugs and subsidizing of doctors' education should also be considered.

Modern medicine is not a science but is the application of science

CHAPTER 8

IS MEDICINE A SCIENCE? WHY IT MATTERS

Changing Medicine to Control Long-Term Costs and Making Medicine Safer

"Medicine is a science of uncertainty and an art of probability,"- William Osler

This book would not be complete without exploring answers to a few more questions. Even after implementing the system suggested in Chapters 6 and 7, we must ensure that we have a sustainable system that encourages safe medicine and keeps long-term costs under control. To achieve this goal, it would help if we had a better understanding about how much of modern medicine is a science and how much its practices are influenced by incentives. We can use this understanding to make medicine less expensive and less hazardous in the future.

Many people regard medicine as science, in the same way that they regard physics or chemistry as sciences. Because of this widespread belief, most people cannot visualize a world without medicine as we know it. This widespread belief has acted as a barrier to a switch-over to medicine that is fundamentally different, less reliant on drugs and surgeries and significantly cheaper and safer.

So, whether medicine is a science, is a question that needs to be explored in more detail. If modern medicine is indeed a science, then we are stuck with the treatments, drugs, and procedures that have already been developed. In science there can be only one truth, so for any given illness there can be only one possible scientific treatment that is best under a given situation. However, if medicine is not a science, we can hope to redevelop it and fill the medical repertoire with a different set of treatments and cures that are more effective, cheaper, and safer.

Is Medicine a Science?

It is true that modern medicine is based on science and that doctors are well versed in the basic biological sciences such as biology, biochemistry, cell biology, and anatomy. But, is modern medicine truly a science in the same sense as are the sciences such as physics, chemistry, microbiology or cell biology? What is the difference between these sciences and medicine?

The answers become clear when we note that modern medicine is only concerned with the *application* of scientific knowledge. Medicine is chiefly concerned with *using* the knowledge discovered by biological scientists to develop treatments and cures. The job of scientists is to discover the truths about nature by revealing its incontrovertible laws. In science, there can be only one truth.

But once these laws are known, the job of a scientist ends and the job of a doctor begins. Since medicine concerns itself with using this knowledge to find techniques to heal people, multiple pathways are usually possible for treating the same disease. For example, if a patient has a heart problem, several healing techniques such as surgery, angioplasty, prescription drugs, non-prescription drugs, and garlic, can all be useful. Similarly, a typical cancer patient might have multiple treatment choices–such as surgery, radiation, or chemotherapy.

Thus, the medical field gives doctors considerable leeway in what treatment to use. Choosing from among these techniques involves tradeoffs between various risks and potential benefits. Judgment and the professional *opinion* of a doctor play a role. This is where medicine becomes more of an *art* than a *science*.

This is also where financial *incentives* of a doctor can play a role. If medicine were a science, then it would be possible to determine with absolute certainty what treatment is best for a given patient *under given circumstances*. There would be no need for a medical opinion or judgment. Every doctor would arrive at the same recommendation. It would not matter if you obtained a second or third opinion. All opinions by all doctors would always be the same.

Under such circumstances, every doctor would always be obligated to use the same treatment, no matter how much or how little money he or she made from it. But such is clearly not the case. Anyone who has been to several doctors for the same disease knows that opinions and recommendations from different doctors can vary widely.

Not only do the doctors exercise judgment in their daily

practice of medicine and their financial incentives play a role, but the situation is more egregious than that. Practices, by large number of doctors with similar perverse incentives over a long period of time, can even corrupt the body of medical knowledge. We will see how this can happen.

The Role of Incentives in Shaping Medical Knowledge

Consider a group of 100 doctors practicing medicine under the same system, so that they all have the same set of incentives. Let us say 5 percent of them are extremely honest and that they always put the patient's interest before their own financial interest. However, the other 95 percent, though not outright dishonest, might be swayed by financial incentives to use treatments that are risky but pay more.

Under such a scenario, it is unlikely that the practices of those 5 percent will gain much acceptance within the medical community. Unfortunately, in medicine, no lab can test the efficacy of a treatment for *every* individual. Every one of the 7 billion humans on earth is different. The response to a given treatment is different for different patients because of the variations in individual physiology.

Thus, the delivery of medicine is based on professional opinion, which under such a scenario will likely be influenced by the 95 percent of less conscientious doctors just because there are more of them.

Thus, in the absence of good ways to test the efficacy and risks of treatments, the practice of medicine is based on *opinion*. The opinion shared by the majority of practitioners becomes the medical standard. The standard treatments get recorded in the medical books, which are considered authoritative sources. In turn, these books are used to train the next generation of doctors. The doctors practicing medicine today have access to this repertoire of treatments because these treatments were developed in the past based on the incentives that existed in the past.

What Happens When a Body of Science Is Corrupted?

The consequences arising from a corrupted body of knowledge can be very serious. Many doctors start to believe in their own medicine, thinking that it is a science. Unaware of the role that incentives have played in the development of medical knowledge, they practice this medicine on themselves and their loved ones. Many will not even consider alternative forms of treatment, even if the patient in front of them is dying.

The system becomes resistant to change. It takes a lot of courage for a doctor to take a different healing approach than the one recommended in the medical texts. In addition, our system employs third parties for payment. If a doctor wants to try a treatment different from the one considered standard, he or she might have trouble getting paid by the insurance company.

There is yet another reason why a doctor must adhere to standard medical practices: fear of malpractice lawsuits. A doctor who tries to deviate from accepted practices risks losing the legal battle in the event he or she is sued for malpractice. In the courtroom, the doctor's actions will be judged by how closely he or she followed established medical standards, even if those standards were developed under perverse incentives.

An example of how these unproven but profitable techniques manage to move into the medical repertoire is the routine performance of procedures such as tonsillectomies. Tonsillectomies remove vital immune system organs because they get swollen while performing their function. An alternative, and better, approach might be simply to advise the patient that the patient's diet (or environment) contains foods or other elements that the body recognizes as toxins and the patient should experiment with avoidance of certain foods (or environmental elements) till the problem goes away. In most cases, the latter suggestion would work for patients and would be appropriate.

But, if most doctors (say 90 percent) start performing tonsillectomies as the preferred treatment, then the practice will become standard medicine. Unless some drastic counter-evidence emerges to indicate the harm done by the procedure, it will continue to be performed by the next generation of doctors. (Tonsils were a problem for me in my childhood, but I never had them removed. The problem has gone away, and in the process I have learned to avoid certain foods.)

Why do People Think of Medicine as a Science?

Most people are aware of the controversial opinions that exist in medicine. They are also aware of the changing nature of many medical opinions. This is unlike true sciences, where natural laws do not change but stay the same from century to century. Yet, despite this evidence, many people continue to put their trust in medicine in the same way as they do in physics,chemistry, or biology.

So why is the general public confused about this concept? One reason for the confusion might be that doctors do have considerable education in the underlying sciences on which medicine is based. Since medicine is practiced by people trained in science, people think it must be science.

Another characteristic that gives medicine an appearance of being scientific is the extensive use of technology in performing medical procedures. The use of high-tech instruments such as X-rays, CAT scan or PET scan machines give the impression that medicine must be science.

It is important to note that these technologies are not medicine. Their use does not turn medicine into science. Use of these machines does not imply advanced understanding of the human body. Though doctors use these machines, in most cases they were not even invented by doctors and, therefore, do not signify greater understanding of the disease process.

Expensive technology is used in medicine because large sums of money are available for payment through the system that involves insurance companies. Though some machines, such as imaging technologies (X-ray, CAT scans and PET scans) provide images of internal body organs, they can also harm the body by subjecting the body to radiation and increasing the risk of diseases such as cancer.

Even after subjecting the body to risk, the images obtained by these machines are often fuzzy and need interpretation by a radiologist. Even expert interpretation of the images can be wrong. Thus, despite the use of expensive technology, there is room for being wrong in diagnosis.

Heavy use of these machines in America does not mean that American doctors understand the human body and disease processes any better than doctors in other countries where there is lesser use of these machines. It does create the impression that medicine is scientific, but it is merely a matter of appearances. Still, to many people, it is enough to make them believe that medicine must be a science.

Another possible reason for the confusion is that some people draw a parallel between medicine and technology. Just as technology evolves and *changes* from year to year, they accept *changing opinions* in medicine as an evolution of knowledge. But note that *technology is not a science*, either. Medicine is application of science, so is technology.

Just as a doctor can heal you by using either garlic or open-heart surgery, so can an engineer design a car to run on either gasoline or electricity. Both the doctor and engineer make use of incontrovertible scientific knowledge discovered by scientists. But, they both have a choice in how to solve a given problem.

To make money, an engineer must design a product in the *least* expensive way so it is affordable for the maximum number of people. Doctors, on the other hand, work with one patient at a time and get paid by insurance. They must choose the *most* expensive procedure, often involving expensive high-tech equipment, in order to make more money. They know their patient is in need and insulated from most of the cost.

What is Scientific Medicine?

Medicine that involves the use of high-tech machines is not necessarily scientific medicine. Some low-tech cures and treatments can be scientific. Scientific medicine consists of treatments based on information so clear and incontrovertible, that it produces cures *almost* 100 percent of the time after such treatment is administered. Not surprisingly, many such cures and treatments were discovered before we started using insurance to pay for treatments.[70]

Remember the discovery of vitamin C to cure scurvy, the discovery of vitamin B1 to cure beriberi, vitamin D to cure rickets, or the discovery of quinine for the treatment of malaria? Substances to cure these diseases were administered in a very low-tech way. The administration was usually by mouth.

Often the substances were made a part of the diet. Yet, the results were miraculous, with *nearly* 100 percent of the patients benefiting from them. These critical discoveries were truly scientific and benefited the human race while relieving much suffering. Those are the types of results we would expect from medicine if today's medicine were truly scientific.

Contrast these cures with today's treatments. Many treatments used today can last for a very long time. Much of the medicine of today *treats*, but does not *cure*. Consider procedures such as bone marrow transplants for cancer, or heart surgery. Such treatments are so expensive and dangerous that they result in costs ranging between $360,000 to $800,000 and *kill* a percentage of the people to whom they are administered.[71]

Treatments such as these make a lot of money for the doctors and hospitals. They require the use of high-tech equipment that seems impressive. But, they subject patients to risk often greater than the risk posed by disease itself.

Even though the ensuing benefit is very small, there is a chance that the follow-up medical treatment will go on for a long time, possibly for life. This will guarantee a long-term income for doctors and hospitals, but the patient will be enslaved to the medical profession.

Other Consequences of Believing that Medicine is a Science

The misunderstanding that modern medicine is a science is causing suffering not only for Americans, but for people all over the world. Because of this misunderstanding, doctors in many poor countries all over the world continue to allow people to die because modern drugs are not available.

They assume that if patented drugs recognized by modern medicine are not used to treat a disease, then no other effective alternative exists. These doctors never try potentially effective treatments from other systems of medicine or herbal medicines that are cheap, readily available, and for which the data about their efficacy is readily available in research journals and on the internet.

Doctors trained in the techniques of modern medicine are usually not able to think of remedies outside of what they have learned in their medical texts and thus might be allowing preventable deaths to occur.

By assuming that all known scientific healing methods exist only in the domain of modern medicine as it is being practiced today, and by ignoring other known effective cures and treatments, doctors might be allowing needless suffering to occur. It would, indeed, be a great tragedy if this is happening today with high frequency in poorer countries that cannot afford the high cost of modern medical drugs. Even many Americans could be suffering because of this same misunderstanding.

Modern Medicine and Alternative Medicine

Modern medicine is not the only type of medicine available in our country or in other nations. Other forms of medicine, such as: herbal medicine, traditional Chinese medicine, Ayurvedic medicine, homeopathy, and so forth are also practiced in the United States and in other countries. However, the prevailing view among most Americans and educated people all over the world is that only modern medicine is true medicine.

I do not consider myself qualified to comment on the efficacy of most of the systems of medicine I just mentioned, although the fact that many of these systems have been practiced for centuries leads me to believe that they must have some merit.

However, there is one exception: herbal medicine. Even though it is currently ignored by practitioners of modern medicine, this type of medicine is just as scientific as modern medicine. The efficacy of herbs has been studied in universities and research institutions throughout the world. The results of these studies are well documented in research journals. What is even more important is that most of this information is readily available on the internet, and often free of cost. Yet, practitioners of modern medicine ignore this type of medicine and do not even consider it modern medicine.

The public thinks that the reason herbal medicine is being ignored is because it is ineffective, or that possibly more research is needed to find more effective herbs.

Policymakers share in this belief. They want to divert more research dollars into this area. They are blissfully unaware that the reason why herbal medicine is being ignored is not because of a dearth of information but because of perverse incentives of doctors.

Because of the false widespread belief, that more research is needed in the area, the National Center for Complementary and Alternative Medicine (NCCAM)*, was established as a part of the National Institutes of Health (NIH) in October of 1998. The establishment of this institute and other such programs presumes that once sufficient research is available, doctors would automatically start using it in their practice. But policymakers are missing the point. No amount of research will bring herbal medicine into the mainstream, unless incentives for doctors are first changed.

Can Evidence-Based Medicine Significantly Lower Healthcare Costs?

During the course of the public debate that preceded the passage of the Affordable Care Act of 2010, in one of his speeches President Obama recommended moving the healthcare system toward the practice of Evidence-Based Medicine (EBM). In fact, the Affordable Care Act provides

---

*As of December 17, 2014, it was renamed 'National Center for Complementary and Integrative Health (NCCIH)'.

funding for EBM by mandating national comparative outcomes research (36, 37). Some readers might also be tempted to think that the practice of evidence-based medicine might produce cheaper and more effective medicine and *resolve the problems* of our healthcare system.

But, the discussion below shows that even evidence-based medicine cannot solve the problems that have been created by *perverse incentives.*

What is Evidence-Based Medicine?

The term *evidence-based medicine* is relatively new. It was first used in 1992 in a paper published in the *Journal of the American Medical Association* (JAMA) (36) to refer to the use of evidence in evaluating the effectiveness of medical techniques, and the use of this evidence in medical decision-making. As you can guess, before the introduction of the term, most Americans were not even aware that the medicine administered by their doctors was not based on clear evidence, no matter how expensive or how risky the medicine was.

Unfortunately, decisions regarding which medical techniques to use on a given patient are based on incentives, and opinion, not on evidence. In the United States, most of the time, treatments are performed by the same doctor who gave the medical opinion in the first place. Thus, doctors have an incentive to recommend the most expensive treatment that they know how to perform.

Since the Affordable Care Act mandates national EBM research (37), it is likely that once the research has been conducted, data will become available to improve the practice of medicine. But how much improvement can we expect?

There is more than one reason why such an approach is likely to fall short of our needs. Let's start by focusing on one area– drug research. A limited form of evidence-based research has been conducted for some time in this area (although the term is generally not used in this context). How well has evidence-based medicine performed in this area?

Evidence-Based Medicine to Evaluate the Effectiveness of Drugs

Drug companies are required to conduct controlled trials on human beings before their drugs can be marketed. This, in a limited sense, is an example of evidence-based research. Much has been made of this type of research, and double-blind studies have been touted as 'scientific'. But a thoughtful reader will note that studies like these do not add anything to the understanding of the underlying mechanisms that make a drug work.

On the contrary, these studies represent an admission by researchers that the mechanism by which these drugs act is too complex to understand completely. Therefore, instead of trying to understand the underlying mechanisms, efforts are focused on gathering *statistical evidence* for their effectiveness.

The studies only tell us if a drug can be effective for some people in a given population and the side effects it can have on that group. Often, the studies do not provide any clue as to what *type of person* the drug will help, or what side effects the drug will have on the person it helps.

In case of drug research, the studies are further skewed by the financial interests of the drug companies (38). Often these studies *understate* the side effects and *overstate* the benefits of a given drug.

Shortcomings of Statistical Evidence

Even if we assume that the drug studies have been conducted honestly, the problems with the results remain because these studies only provide statistical evidence. The results apply only to populations, not individuals. Transferring these statistical results to individuals in the population can be disastrous.

Consider, for example, a drug that a pharmaceutical company tests on 1,000 patients who suffer from a particular medical condition. Let's say the drug proves helpful to 600 patients, but harms the other 400. The drug company could market the drug as being 60 percent effective. A doctor might even prescribe it to you, saying that it is 60 percent effective. However, it might turn out that your body physiology is similar to those 400 patients who were harmed by the drug. In this case, the treatment could prove harmful to you, even though it has been "scientifically" proven to be 60 percent effective.

The Biggest Limitation of Evidence-Based Medicine

There is yet another reason why evidence-based medicine cannot solve all our cost or quality problems. All evidence-based research can do is compare two or more treatments from *available* techniques within the medical repertoire. These treatments, whether they are drugs or surgical techniques, have been developed by our healthcare system (and similar systems around the world) under a given set of incentives.

Collectively, we refer to these as "modern medicine." The research into evidence-based medicine assumes that these treatments, techniques, and drugs are *science*. i.e. no other available techniques from alternative medicine are effective.

Research into evidence-based medicine ignores the role of incentives in the development of this body of knowledge. Instead, the researchers assume that these drugs or treatments were developed and standardized solely because they were the best, most cost-effective ways of treating patients.

Evidence-based medicine then proceeds to pick out the best possible treatments from this collection. It completely *ignores* treatments that might be extremely effective and safe but have never been accepted by modern medicine simply because they were *so safe and inexpensive* that the skills of a practitioner were not needed to administer them.

The body of knowledge we call *modern medicine* is incomplete and misses such cheaper and safer treatments. By ignoring the role of incentives in the development of medicine and awarding the status of science to present medicine, we will continue to run into similar problems regarding the cost and safety of medicine that have plagued us for the last several decades. Moreover, the research into evidence-based medicine is not enough to resolve *"The Final Paradox of Healthcare Costs."*

The Final Paradox of Healthcare Costs

Some people believe that it is futile to try making people healthy to save on national healthcare costs, because as the health of a population increases, so does the life span of individuals in that population. Thus, the number of elderly in the population also increases. Since the elderly consume more healthcare dollars, more people living longer will *increase* healthcare costs. Thus, they believe, a healthier and longer-living population can actually *raise* total national healthcare costs, not lower them.

Why Does the Paradox Exist?

Let us see why this paradox exists and how the system described in Chapters 6 and 7 can lead to a new paradigm for the practice of medicine and thus resolve this paradox, too.

The paradox only exists because of another quirk in our healthcare system. Apart from the fact that our system delivers medicine through a business model, the providers in the system benefit from 'disease' rather than 'health.' Although we call our system a 'healthcare system,' this is a misnomer. Our healthcare system has actually evolved into a form of *commerce based on disease*. A better characterization would be *disease-care* system. Because it is also a for-profit system, its practitioners have a motive to sell more medicine to sick people.

In the United States, the elderly provide a lucrative market for healthcare services because they are more likely to be anxious about their health. Even if they do not need medicine and their symptoms are the result of the normal aging process, they can easily be persuaded to use more medicine. They are also covered by a good health insurance under Medicare.

As long as we have a *disease-care* system in combination with a lucrative market for private providers, provided by the elderly, this paradox cannot be resolved.

If we want to discourage practitioners from pushing more medicine, we must abandon the present method of private for-profit practitioners being paid by the fee-for-service method because these practitioners benefit from disease. By changing the system as outlined in Chapters 6 and 7, we can expect the system to eventually become less focused on delivering treatments for *sickness* and more focused on creating health. We can also expect practitioners in the system to start encouraging *prevention* rather than developing more expensive methods for *treating* diseases.

If we want a way out of this paradox, two things need to happen in our healthcare system. First, the focus of our healthcare system needs to shift to the encouragement of prevention rather than to *disease-care*. Second, the methods employed to treat disease also need to change.

If we want to make medicine drastically cheaper and safer, we need to move to a system that employs foods, herbs, and lifestyle changes as treatments instead of drugs, surgeries, and radiation as the preferred treatments. Only then can we expect our elderly to live long lives without placing an excessive cost burden on the system.

It is quite clear that the current system does not encourage prevention. Although doctors and other professionals might pay lip-service to prevention, they realize that ultimately it will not help their earnings if most of the diseases can be prevented and, thus, the need for medical services is reduced.

Even when doctors (and dentists) encourage prevention, they encourage it through regular checkups and intervention, which require their services. These checkups give doctors (and dentists) opportunities for generating more business.

By convincing otherwise healthy patients of the risk of contracting disease in the *future*, doctors can easily convince their patients that they need treatment *now*. Doctors routinely under-emphasize the harm that their treatments can do.

While prevention is the best method of staying healthy, despite one's best efforts, not everyone can always prevent every disease. As a society, we will always be in need of some medicine. Only the availability of much cheaper and safer medicines can help our elderly to live long and productive lives without burdening the system with excessive costs. Availability and development of this type of medicine will require a change in incentives, rather than simply choosing the best from whatever medicine has been developed under the current system.

Evidence suggests that long life is possible without medical intervention with modern techniques, since many long-living cultures do *not* depend on doctors for their health as much as Americans do (39), (40).

What is Good about Modern Medicine?

Although incentives built into its payment system are responsible for modern medicine's shortcomings, this medicine also has some strengths. All systems have variables, some good, others bad. Because our *sickness-care* system encourages risky medicine, it has also developed some strengths as unintended consequences.

One such strength is that the techniques and skills developed under our system (which encourages more risky practices) can be very useful in *critical care*. For example, if one were to suffer a serious accident where chances of living were slim, modern medicine could come to one's rescue. In such situations, safer medicine (such as herbal medicine) might not be of much use and the risk of not doing anything could exceed the risk of treatment using methods that might be deemed unsafe in other situations.

American doctors (as well as doctors in other countries) have succeeded in rescuing patients from near-death situations.[72] When this happens, doctors can gain a hero's status; sometimes gaining as much popularity as the people in showbiz. This type of media attention tends to overemphasize the triumphs of modern medicine while ignoring its myriad shortcomings.

Such *occasional* triumphs in no way compensate for the thousands who *routinely* die each year under our system as a result of medical mistakes that largely occur because our system encourages unsafe medicine. Nor can we ignore the pain caused by bankruptcies resulting from medical bills, even in cases when medicine has been able to help. Inflated medical bills can spell financial ruin for patients, even when medicine saves their lives.

Another often-offered justification for not changing our system is that the very high income of doctors encourages more academically bright students into the profession. Unfortunately, this need for bright doctors arises *only* because the system encourages *unsafe* medicine that requires greater skill to practice. If our system were designed properly, it would not encourage risky medicine and highly skilled doctors would not be needed. I would rather be treated by a doctor with average skill using a safe treatment rather than by a highly skilled doctor using a risky treatment. Allowing one's health to depend on the skill of a surgeon, where a slip of the knife could make the difference between life and death, is not the kind of medicine one should seek.

As we mentioned previously, not every doctor practicing in our system is academically bright. The lure of easy money for doctors in the United States has encouraged the opening of medical schools in the Caribbean and elsewhere in the world, which exist for the sole purpose of awarding medical degrees so that graduates of these schools can practice in the United States.

Applicants rejected from U.S. medical schools can easily enter these medical schools because of lax admission requirements. Not all these schools are eligible for U.S. student loans, but as long as one has money to pay the tuition, it is relatively easy. On graduation, the graduates must pass an exam before they can practice in the United States, but the bar has now been lowered. Once in the system, they can make as much money as any other doctor because of our healthcare system's faulty business model.

The present system also wastes talent. Since there is less money to be made in medical research than in the practice of medicine, the talent is attracted to the practice of medicine rather than research. The skills of academically bright students might be better used in research, but the system does not encourage or reward it.

All systems have some good points and some bad. It is impossible to have an excellent system without some flaws. On the other hand, even a bad system such as ours can produce some good results. The good features of our system are unintended consequences resulting from an otherwise inflation-prone and hazardous system. The fact that our system *can* produce better results in critical care should not be a reason to keep it. Many of the skills needed in critical care could continue to be developed and improved even in the changed system proposed in this book.

Some people are afraid that if incentives are changed, medical research will stop. These fears are also baseless. If we switch to a better system of incentives, there will continue to be innovation in medicine, but now for the right reasons. Procedures will now not be developed simply because they are *profitable* to the providers, but because they are *beneficial* to the patient.

Changed incentives for the doctors will lead to a new perception of health in our society. We have a disease-care system that encourages the belief that people need the help of disease-care professionals to be healthy (and thus, to avoid them). Regular health checkups, regular mammograms, and drugs to decrease the risk factors have been encouraged by the professionals, while the risk of intervention following these checkups has been downplayed. An incorrect impression – that to live a long life, medical intervention is necessary – has been created.

The truth is that excessive medical intervention decreases life, because under the present incentive system it is necessarily risky. My close relatives have lived well into their nineties with virtually no medical intervention. They died peacefully in their homes, without any end-of-life care.

Our goal as a society should be for people to live to be a hundred without medical intervention, and then die in their sleep.[73] However, such a *vision is being hidden from us by a system* that benefits from tremendous profits that can be generated by providing end-of-life healthcare using Medicare dollars.

Often, heroic efforts are made to save the lives of patients toward the end of their lives (sometimes against their wishes), all in the name of respect for life. *The healthcare providers never like to mention the fact that these heroic efforts also generate huge profits for them.*

Society's Views on Medicine.

In our society, many people believe that drugs, surgeries and other medical interventions are necessary to be disease-free. Many more people believe that medical checkups and other assistance of doctors is the only way to remain healthy. These views are not accurate and have been instilled into us by the medical providers who have a natural interest in keeping people dependent on them. Such views on health in our society will not change unless we change the system.

One often overlooked characteristic of a market-based economy is that the very people who are experts in their fields– and thus capable of changing society's views–are usually the individuals who are also *engaged in profiting from the markets.*

It is in their interest to mold the views of society in ways that allow them to continue to profit from these markets. It is in their interest to propagate views that keep people dependent on them. Unless we first change the system, we cannot expect experts to teach the public about self-reliance in the area of health.

Similarly, there will also be some minor shortcomings in our new system, if we adopt a mostly government-run system as suggested in Chapters 6 and 7. With very few doctors in private practice, doctors on salaries will have no incentive to shape societal views either way. In that case, the government will have to fill in the void. *Government institutions would have to step in and provide authentic, unbiased, and non-controversial information* about health and prevention, a rarity today.

A New Paradigm of Medicine

By switching to the new system, we will eventually create a new paradigm for the practice of medicine–a system that encourages prevention rather than medical intervention.

Let us also hope that doctors in this system would first try safer treatments and cures before resorting to riskier practices such as prescription medications or surgeries. Then, what we call *alternative* medicine today will become the *mainstream* medicine of tomorrow. Let us hope we will all be able to live one-hundred years of a full, productive life without medical intervention, and then die peacefully in our sleep.

Adding a totally free system with salaried doctors to our existing system would be a good place to begin this change. In the long run, we might want to restrict fee-for-service medicine only to those who can pay for it out-of-pocket.

Conclusion

Modern medicine need not consist of unsafe and expensive treatments such as surgeries or prescription drugs. Effective treatments found in herbal medicine or other alternative forms of medicine can be incorporated into modern medicine if doctors' incentives are changed. Also, increasing the life span of people need not necessarily result in increased healthcare costs, as long as prevention and the administration of cheaper medicine is encouraged.

The excessive lawsuits in our system are just another consequence of a system that encourages unsafe medicine.

CHAPTER 9

MEDICAL MALPRACTICE REFORM

When we reform our healthcare system as outlined in the previous chapters, malpractice costs will go down. Malpractice suits will be reduced by changing to safer medicine.[74] There would be no need to put arbitrary limits on malpractice awards that might deny justice to some deserving patients while encouraging complacency for the doctors. Thus, there would be no need to alter our legal system to help our faulty healthcare system. Once the incentives for doctors are altered, the healthcare system will be safer and able to stand on its own without any aid from a *modified* legal system. By the end of this chapter, readers will realize that malpractice suits are *just another consequence* of our faulty healthcare system.

Lawsuits need not be artificially curbed. Their existence is *evidence* of the shortcomings in our system. Under the solution that has been proposed in this book, there could still be a need for financial compensation in rare cases, but it would be comparatively small and could be met without resorting to lawsuits (as will be explained later in the chapter).

The changes to our healthcare system must first be made before we consider alternative ways for compensating the medically injured. To understand why we have so many lawsuits in our system we must understand the underlying reasons.

Conventional Wisdom about Malpractice Suits

The Common Moral Argument

A popular explanation for the large number of lawsuits in America is that Americans are inherently litigious people. We are told that we Americans are not fair people and sue the very doctors who are trying to save our lives. It is generally accepted that this attitude is unfair to doctors who work very hard to help their patients but must also face the potential of lawsuits from these same patients who they are trying to help. Proponents of tort reform, therefore, argue that it is perfectly justified to limit the liability of doctors when they accidentally injure their patients in the process of healing them.

They also argue that as a bonus, tort reform will also lower the costs of medicine since doctors can now afford to charge less.

Let us examine the validity of the first argument. (the answer to the second argument has been discussed in Chapter 2 and 4, where I showed that doctors have no incentive to compete on price).

Are we a Litigious Society?

Societies are not inherently litigious. They are neither good nor evil. Just as we Americans do not pay our doctors more than in other countries because we are a more generous society, we do not sue more because we are a litigious society. The system under which people live determines their collective behavior. In other words, even though some people might think that Americans are inherently litigious people, this collective behavior is the result of peculiarities in our healthcare and legal environments. Elements present in these environments result in large numbers of malpractice suits. Let us examine these.

Reasons for Large Numbers of Medical Malpractice Lawsuits in America

Risky Medicine Involving Surgeries and Prescriptions

The foremost reason for the large number of lawsuits is that our present system of payment encourages the practice of risky medicine. This fact, discussed throughout the book, needs no further elaboration. Going to a doctor should inspire hope. Yet, many people when going to a doctor are also afraid. Many people expect that the treatment would involve prescription drugs or surgery. Both of these are unsafe.

Modern medicine has treatments for many diseases but few cures, so most people do not even expect complete recovery. Whether the treatment turns out to be a drug or surgery, they expect to put up with some of its damaging side effects.

Risk is the hallmark of modern medicine. It is this feature that distinguishes modern medicine from alternative systems of medicine. The medical profession has been able to convince patients that medicine based on drugs and surgeries is true medicine even if it involves risk because such medicine is "scientific." Any other type of medicine even when it achieves better results is dubbed as quackery just because it is safer.

So it should not surprise anyone that riskier treatments will result more lawsuits.

Delivery of Medicine Through a Business Model

Risky medicine is not the only reason for the large number of lawsuits under our system. Our system turns doctors into *businessmen and businesswomen.* Doctors while making money must also show that they are doing what is best for the patient *regardless* of their financial interests.

These conflicting requirements imposed on them: one by the incentive system and the other by the expectations of the society, forces them to be subtle. *Occasionally, patients see through this illusion* and may sense that their health is not the priority of their doctor. They may get the impression that the doctor's financial interests are playing a greater role in their treatment, thus creating an atmosphere of *distrust.*

Many lawsuits result from distrust. You cannot blame the patients for their anger if they are led to believe that everything is being done only for their benefit even though their doctors are delivering medicine through a business model.

Expensive Medicine

Not only is the present system the *cause* of high prices but the *high prices in turn are a factor in the rising number of malpractice lawsuits.* The super high prices of medicine can raise the expectations of some patients. Patients are used to dealings in free markets. In free markets, high prices are a sign of quality. The huge medical bills that patients encounter, therefore, might raise the expectations of some patients.

Some patients conclude that the medical system that costs so much must be able to perform miracles. To be able to make so much money doctors must be superhuman. This could raise their expectations about what they can expect from their doctors. When these patients visit their doctor, the expectation might be that their doctor will be perfect in diagnosis and treatment. If these expectations are not met, it can trigger lawsuits. Lawsuits that arise from the missed or misdiagnosis generally fall in this category.[75]

No Mechanism for Automatic Compensation for Medical Injuries

Unlike the Workers' Compensation program where if workers get injured on the job they are automatically compensated for injuries without having to sue the employer, our medical system does not have any such mechanism.

Our system is unfair to the patients because injured patients badly need financial compensation. For the most part, compensation is needed just to pay for additional medical bills that will result from the injury that has already been caused. Most patients are in a severely physically weakened condition due to medical injuries. In addition, they are now required to navigate the legal maze just to get compensation for their injuries. The circumstances of most people do not permit them to take legal action and many simply accept their suffering.

However a small number, *about 2 percent of the medically injured patients do sue*. Modern medicine has become so risky, and the number of injuries in medicine is so large that *even* such a small percentage of people suing results in a large number of lawsuits.

In most industrialized countries, some form of government body compensates the medically injured. The medicine in most countries is also free so that any further medical expenses are paid by the system, reducing the need to sue.

Why don't we such a system in America? For answer to this question see section entitled *'Medicine as a Failed Business'* later in this chapter.

Faith in the Legal System

Last but not the least, people in America are litigious because they have *faith* in their legal system. The number of lawsuits in any country is not solely dependent on how many people are suffering. It also depends upon whether people have faith in their legal system. In countries where the legal system is so inefficient that even simple cases take years or even decades to decide, few bother to sue.

In the United States, we have a reasonably good civil legal system[76] capable of deciding cases quickly (compared to many other countries of the world). So it encourages *more* lawsuits.

Also in tort cases, U.S. lawyers can work on contingency basis, and do not require the client to put money up front. This encourages more lawsuits but is also a good thing because without this provision, the poor would not be able to obtain compensation when injured.

Another benefit of a contingency-based system is that it *discourages frivolous lawsuits* because lawyers often must spend tens of thousands of dollars of their own money before they can take the case to the courtroom. Therefore, they do not like to accept cases that are without merit.

Arguments for Limiting Medical Malpractice Damages

Instead of examining the reasons why many medical malpractice suits occur in our society, some people have argued for modifying our legal system to aid our healthcare system.

Some believe that in order to pay for the high malpractice insurance, doctors must keep their prices higher. This belief follows from the *false assumption that the healthcare market is a free market*. In free markets, providers compete with each other on prices. We have already discussed the fallacies of this argument in Chapter 4.

In our system the consumer is shielded from the price through a system of insurance and co-pays, so *doctors do not have to lower their prices* to stay in business. Chapter 4, showed how doctors can actually *increase* their business by raising their prices. Therefore they would have no motivation to lower prices even if their expenses were lowered.

Some people argue that the extra tests doctors order to cover themselves against lawsuits are raising costs. There is some truth in this argument, although if medicine were safer, it would reduce the need for extra testing.

During the presidency of George W. Bush, the subject of medical malpractice was brought up so often by the President that most Americans now mistakenly believe that malpractice problem is contributing to the price spiral. Since the general public does not have an in-depth understanding of our healthcare system, it is reasonable that many Americans will believe in this fallacy.

It is also quite understandable why the doctors and their malpractice insurance companies would support such a position. Like any other professionals, doctors do not want to be sued. It is in their interest to use any reasoning that the public would *buy* to lower their liability as well as their malpractice insurance premiums.

The malpractice issue serves as a red herring to cause even more confusion in the already confused minds of the public. But, as consumers of healthcare, readers of this book must be on guard against false arguments.

Texas Constitutional Amendment to Limit Malpractice Damages

A very good illustration of the effects of limiting the liability for doctors is provided by examining what happened in Texas in 2003. The story of Texas provides a window into what effect limiting of malpractice awards would have if this type of reform were carried out at national level.[77]

In 2003, when George W. Bush was president, the insurance companies and the doctors in Texas sensed the mood of the people. Because of the repeated public statements by the President, people had started to believe that the malpractice lawsuits were the true cause of inflation in medicine. It was a unique opportunity for insurance companies and the doctors to do something about the problem. In the White House, a president who had been the governor of Texas, was solidly in favor of this type of malpractice reform. Sensing the opportunity, the medical interests in Texas launched their campaign. They introduced Proposition 12, a constitutional Amendment to the Texas constitution that would limit the liability of doctors in malpractice cases.

Spending millions, these interests mailed brochures containing pictures of smiling babies and stating that the delivery of babies was suffering in rural Texas because there were simply no doctors to deliver them. They said this was the fault of the malpractice system. They said too many greedy lawyers were making it difficult for doctors and it was no longer economically feasible to practice in the rural areas. Even though the campaign was based on misstated facts and half-truths, it was an easy sell. People do not understand the intricacies of healthcare markets and therefore hold many untrue notions. Proposition 12 passed.

Many years later, all the problems in Texas remain. Malpractice insurance premiums have fallen slightly making it more attractive for doctors to practice in Texas. Doctors are moving in from other states and the state board has had its hands full issuing new licenses. However, these doctors did not move to the rural areas of Texas but are moving to wealthy suburbs of Dallas and Houston. That is where the *money* is. The medical costs are not going *down* but are going *up*. In fact, Texas was transformed into a state with one of the fastest rising healthcare costs.[78]

To the readers of this book, the story of Texas should not come as a surprise. It should be obvious that malpractice limits are not going to control costs. But why are medical costs in Texas *rising*? The section below will attempt to answer that question.

Some Cost-Lowering Effects of Malpractice Lawsuits

Malpractice lawsuits have often been blamed for raising the cost of medicine. But can the threat of lawsuits *lower* medical costs?

Insurance, fee-for-service payments to doctors, and the patients' propensity for getting back part of what they pay to insurance companies–all encourage *more* medicine. *Only the threat of lawsuits discourages excessive or unsafe medicine.*

For example, the threat of lawsuits keeps doctors from performing surgeries on older patients who might have little to benefit from surgery but can die from it thus increasing the chance of a malpractice suit. Thus, malpractice suits are a *deterrent* to unnecessary or careless medicine. Since so many incentives in the system encourage *more* medicine we also need a *disincentive*.

We need to keep doctors on their toes if they are going to insist on using so much unsafe medicine. The threat of lawsuits plays an important role in the scheme for reducing the practice of perilous medicine.

One reason why healthcare costs rose in Texas was that the atmosphere became more *lax*. If doctors make more medical mistakes, the lawsuit awards would now be limited mostly to actual damages (Punitive damages were severely limited by the new law). Because the awards were limited, fewer lawyers are willing to take cases from the *poor* and the *old* who cannot show their lawsuits can bring big damage awards. There is now less risk of getting sued by the *poor*, the *old*, the *unemployed* and the *housewives*.

Medicine as a Failed Business

For the malpractice system to be fair to doctors as well as patients, not only do the doctors need protection from unfair lawsuits, but patients also need fair compensation when injured by the system. There needs to be a simple evaluation procedure administered by an impartial agency that fairly compensates the medically injured without patients having the need to sue.

It is unfair to burden sick patients with navigating the legal system to get compensation. *But why don't we already have such a system?* The reason is very simple: if we were to automatically compensate everyone who is injured by the present system then the *cost of such compensation will far exceed the total amount of money that is required to provide universal coverage in America.*

This fact will likely send a chill down the spine of anyone who first learns of it. Our system, the most expensive in the world,is causing so much harm that it cannot even afford to pay for the injuries it is causing! It speaks to the failure of a system designed around perverse incentives to doctors.

Then, why does the system continue to operate? It operates because only 2 percent of the medically injured bother to file a lawsuit. What about the other 98 percent? In their weakened condition, these people do not have the energy or the will to steer through our legal system to obtain justice.

In other words, the only reason that our sick system continues to function is because most injured in the system are willing to accept their misfortune and live with their injuries without asking for compensation.

This fact alone is strong evidence that our healthcare system is *fundamentally* flawed. Instead of mending the system, advocates of limiting malpractice liability inadvertently want to protect it by *further* rewarding the *same* providers whose incentives are causing the *problem*.

Why Will Changing our System Automatically Bring Down Malpractice Costs?

Once we are able to change our healthcare system so that there are no incentives for practicing risky medicine, the medicine will become safer. When we do not pay our doctors more for practicing unsafe medicine, less of it will be practiced. When we do not pay them on a fee-for-service method, fewer unnecessary *services* will be dispensed.

When we do not give incentives to the drug companies for developing patented drugs, all healing substances in nature will be explored including safer natural substances that cannot be patented. When our hospitals are government owned, there will be no profits for the overuse of potentially harmful medical equipment in the hospitals. An all-around practice of safer medicine will thus bring down the number of lawsuits.

Assuming that there will always be some unsafe medicine that would need to be practiced and medical injuries can still occur even under a changed system, we need to make the system fair for everyone by providing an impartial compensating mechanism similar to the workers' compensation system. Not only can such a system help patients by providing them with needed compensation, but it can also bring down the threat of lawsuits for doctors.

Medical Compensation Board

A situation similar to the one we are facing today in our healthcare system, also occurred in the American work environment during the early twentieth century. Because of the lack of safety standards for industries of that time, there were excessive workplace injuries. The injured workers did not have the resources to sue while the injuries also rendered them incapable of earning their livelihood.

In response to the workers' needs, the workers' compensation system evolved (1902-1949). The system has a simplified process for providing compensation to workers who are injured on the job. The workers do not have to go through the more costly, lengthy, and uncertain legal process to receive compensation for their injuries. They can simply go the state workers' compensation office. The compensation is determined by administrative procedure. The payments are usually smaller than what they would be if the workers were to sue in the courts. But, few injured workers bother to sue because it avoids the hassle of going through the legal system. The system provides immediately needed income to the workers.

Employers benefit too, because they do not have to spend time and resources to defend themselves against lawsuits. Instead, employers pay insurance premiums into the workers' compensation fund that covers them against most workers' claims.

The injured workers do not have to accept workers' compensation if they do not wish to. The workers' compensation system in no way impinges on the freedom of workers to sue if they so choose. However, if they choose to sue, they are not entitled to the workers' compensation payments. Thus, the workers' compensation system, because of its simplicity, provides a win-win situation for workers as well as employers.

Since there is no such mechanism for paying out to the medically injured, patients have no other choice but to sue.

Here then are the three ways in which the new healthcare system and a medical board for processing automatic compensations can result in a smaller number of lawsuits.

1. When we change the incentives to providers of the healthcare, there will be no higher payments for riskier procedures; therefore, these will not be performed unnecessarily. Hence, there will be fewer injuries in the system and fewer lawsuits.

2. If everyone is covered by a free healthcare system, then any rare injury occurring in the healthcare system will be less of a financial burden on the injured party because any subsequent medical bills will be covered

by the free healthcare system thus reducing the awards per lawsuit.

3. If we set up a board for the compensation for the medically injured, then there will be less need for lawsuits since damages can quickly be paid by the compensation board.

Conclusion

Although the prevailing view of most Americans is that the lawsuits are the cause of rising healthcare prices, it should be clear to the readers of this book that malpractice lawsuits are a natural consequence of a healthcare system that pays doctors more to deliver riskier medicine. These lawsuits are evidence of a healthcare system incentivized to produce hazardous medicine. A logical solution to solving the malpractice problem is to eliminate the underlying fundamental causes that are resulting in these lawsuits.

A method of change has been proposed earlier in the book. The economic benefits of the change as well as improvement in the quality of healthcare (and the reduction in lawsuits) will probably occur slowly. The doctors have been trained under the old system.The medical treatments for the various illnesses have been developed and practiced under a system of incentives that has been in place since at least the early part ofthe twentieth century. These treatments and practices have become entrenched in medical practice. Even if financial incentives for practicing medicine were changed today, the medicine itself will take longer to change. But this is something we must be willing to put up with.

The United States is inadvertently raising costs in some other countries, such as England. England has to pay higher salaries to their doctors to discourage them from migrating to America.

CHAPTER 10

FREQUENTLY ASKED QUESTIONS

1. If the United States were to provide free healthcare to all its citizens, wouldn't taxes have to be raised for everyone?

Not true. The medical prices in the United States are highly inflated under the present system. If the changes proposed in this book were implemented, it would lower the medical costs to about 40 percent of what they are now. This will reduce the cost to the government to provide the healthcare services it is already providing under the Medicare, Medicaid, and V.A. programs. This will save more than $1.74 trillion dollars every year on these programs, enough to cover all citizens in the country.

2. If the present system of medical payments is not a free-market system, then how do we know what the free-market system prices are?

The free-market prices of healthcare would be prices that doctors, hospitals, and drug companies will be able to charge if our citizens were asked to pay 100 percent of their medical expenses out of pocket, in other words, without using any health insurance money. In 2013, the median household income in the United States was about $52,000. This income is not sufficient to support present-day prices in medicine. Under such a system, the hospitals would not be able to charge around $10,000 per night for a hospital stay as they now do in some large cities. There would be few or no drugs on the market, which cost $50,000 per year or more. Such drugs, if prescribed, would have to be sold at much lower prices. Safer natural substances would have to be used. Knowledge already exists and research has already been undertaken about their safety and effectiveness. Doctors are ignoring these inexpensive therapeutic substances because the use of non-prescription substances requires less reliance on doctors. The fees that doctors charge would also have to be much lower than what they are charging today, and doctors would have to be much more responsive to the needs of their patients.

The type of medicine practiced by doctors would also be different. The medicine would not consist mostly of surgeries such as open-heart surgeries, which can cost upwards of $500,000 in some cities, and are still frequently performed even though many doctors believe they are worthless. Few surgeries of any kind would be performed. Those that are,would be performed at costs that are much lower than rates being charged today. Doctors would not be able to bill insurance companies as they do now, even when a patient dies during a surgery.

3. You say that our system will have to be like the British system. Many Americans do not like the British system because Britain rations healthcare and sometimes you have to wait for non-emergency surgeries.

Under the system that is being proposed in this book, free medicine would be available to everyone who wants it without regard to their income. However, no one would be forced to use the free system if they do not want to. They would have the option to pay for their healthcare through supplemental health insurance just as they do now but at much-reduced prices. If you bought supplemental insurance, then you would not be subject to a wait for your surgery. Because of the availability of an alternate free system, the supplemental health insurance prices would come down for those who do not want their healthcare rationed or who do not want to wait for non-emergency surgeries.

In addition, if you ever face a temporary financial crisis in your life such as a temporary loss of employment and you cannot pay the supplementary insurance premiums, you would not have to worry about going bankrupt in case of an unexpected sickness. The free system will serve as a backup for such situations. People in the lower-income brackets will benefit, too, because they will be able to avail themselves of free healthcare.

4. Does the British government pay less than the medical providers deserve?

No. Just as the best way to determine the fair price of a product is to allow the free markets to fix the price, the best way to determine the incomes of various professionals is to let free markets fix their salaries. Even though the professionals, such as doctors and nurses in England, are paid a salary, their salaries are determined by the laws of supply and demand. Therefore, they are fair salaries. When a shortage of doctors and nurses exists, their salaries go up, which encourages more entrants into the market. Similarly, when there is glut of professionals in this area, the salaries fall.

Even in America, many professionals are employed on a salary only basis. For example, our soldiers, police, teachers, nurses, judges, and professors are paid on a salary basis. This does not mean that they are being paid less than they deserve. Their salaries are determined by the free market laws of supply and demand. In times of shortage of these professionals, their salaries move up and in times of glut, the salaries go down.

Thus, it would neither be unprecedented nor unfair to pay most doctors on a salary basis. In fact, it probably would be a much fairer and more sustainable system than what we have now. The present system is unfair because it makes payments for procedures rather than health. Since unsafe procedures pay more, we are getting unsafe medicine at high prices.

In fact, the healthcare system in America also affects the prices of medicine in England, Canada, and many other countries in the world in more than one way. Because the incomes of doctors in America are unusually high, England must pay British doctors very high salaries; otherwise it would lose its doctors to the United States There are very few barriers for them to migrate to the United States because the medical education is almost the same, and there are no language or cultural barriers between England and the United States.

In addition, many countries of the world look to the United States to provide the lead in technology and healthcare fields. Since most of the medicine being practiced in the United States as well as in the rest of the world is not evidence based, most of the world follows the lead of the United States in various medical practices. Few people in other countries realize that the medicine based on the heavy use of drugs and surgeries is a result of the incentive system in the United States. The practices used in the United States are automatically assumed as being "scientific" by other countries.

5. If we spend less on healthcare, won't we lose innovation in healthcare technology?

Many Americans are proud that U.S. hospitals are equipped with highly sophisticated equipment; they might worry that the healthcare system recommended in this book could discourage innovation. This is a needless worry since little or none of the high-tech equipment in hospitals or doctors' offices has been designed by doctors. The high-tech equipment that is used in medicine has been designed mostly by physicists or electrical engineers. America is home to some of the world's best electrical engineers, physicists, and technical innovators.

Our markets in the areas of electronics are highly competitive. We also have some of the best universities in the world for obtaining technical education. This environment is responsible for producing highly capable scientists, engineers, and innovators. In fact, our technical industries will flourish more if the healthcare prices go down because industries will become more competitive when they do not have to pay high healthcare premiums for their employees.

The use of high-tech equipment in medicine must be kept to a minimum. We are not robots. We are part of nature, and when we use high-tech interventions, they have the potential of doing more harm than good. A lot of the use of high-tech equipment in medicine actually causes disease. For example, the imaging machines such as X-rays and CAT scans subject the body to harmful radiation. Radiation in a single CAT scan can be 50 to 100 times that of a chest X-ray and can actually cause cancer.

6. If doctors were paid on a salary basis, wouldn't they lose their motivation to heal their patients?

The way our system is functioning now, it is very difficult to tell how many people are coming into the medical profession to truly help the sick, and how many people become doctors just because of the money. I believe the new system would be better at attracting only those professionals who truly want to help the sick.

It is better to have a system where there is no extra financial incentives offered for healing (other than the satisfaction that comes from helping people) rather than giving the wrong financial incentives that encourage intervention that can actually hurt the sick.

7. Won't research suffer under the new system?

The present system encourages only the type of research that offers high financial rewards to its practitioners. If there are inexpensive but highly effective methods of treatment available, these are either not pursued or they are suppressed by the providers. The providers have nothing to gain from developing cheaper medicine as long as they know the patients are covered by insurance. They are able to demand astronomical figures from their patients because patients are insulated from the cost.

When it comes to research, our present system is a mixed bag. It only encourages the type of research that can make large sums of money for the providers. At the same time, it discourages investigation into simpler, more effective treatments that might be safer for the patient. The present system is not necessarily helping promote needed research but is getting in the way of developing cheaper and safer methods of treatment.

It is possible to assign the task of medical research to universities and research institutions. Research done in this way will be undertaken to find *all possible* ways of treating diseases rather than focusing only on the *subset* of treatment methods that can make huge sums of money for the medical providers.

8. If we pay doctors salaries only, won't highly skilled surgeons stop being attracted into the system?

When medicine becomes safer, we will not need very highly skilled surgeons. In their place, we would need doctors who are in the profession to genuinely help the sick and can abide by the Hippocratic oath: first do no harm. I would rather be treated by a doctor of average intelligence who cares for me and is willing to suggest safer cures rather than a very intelligent doctor who believes in risky treatments and whose primary goal is to make money.

9. I had a problem with my back, and I tried several alternative medicine techniques that did not help. Finally, I got back surgery that seems to be helping. Doesn't that prove that modern medicine is good and should not be changed?

Nowhere in this book have I implied that modern medicine is not *any* good. There will be times when alternative medicine cures will fail and modern medicine will work. Just as modern medicine is incomplete so is alternative medicine.

Modern medicine is doing some good but a lot of harm. Our system could be made much better and much cheaper if only incentives in it were changed. The changes recommended in this book will not alter the positive side of medicine. They would, however, encourage the practice of medicine that is cheaper and safer. In the present system, doctors are encouraged to intervene in patients' health for their financial gain and provide unsafe treatments because these pay more. We need a system more focused on patients health and less on doctors' pocket-book.

10. Can the United States lower its cost of healthcare below what it costs in Great Britain?

Possibly. The United States is inadvertently raising costs in some other countries, such as England. England has to pay higher salaries to their doctors to discourage them from migrating to America. If the United States switches to a salaried system, both England and the United States might be able to save on doctors' salaries. Costs in both the countries could come down automatically without either country taking any other measures.

Another policy matter we need to consider is abolishing the system of patents for the development of drugs. If we abolish granting drug patents, we can assign the research task to universities or government agencies such as the National Institutes of Health for the few drugs that still might be needed. There will be no motive for these institutions to promote only more expensive alternatives. The present system discourages the use of safer therapeutic substances that have already been studied.

11. Isn't the system that you have recommended social medicine?

I am a believer in free markets and in the capitalistic system. But, if I support such a system, I also have the responsibility to understand *when* and *why* markets work. Free-markets only work when consumers are risking their own money. People also need to be healthy to be able to meaningfully participate in the markets.

Trying to make use of markets for the delivery of healthcare when these conditions are not met can only mean one thing: a problematic system.

In fact, if we do not do anything about it, our *healthcare* system can become a liability for our *capitalistic* system. Recent bankruptcies in the automobile industry have proved that.

These were due in part to high healthcare premiums the employers had to pay, putting them at a competitive disadvantage against similar industries worldwide. The high healthcare costs are also a disincentive to the manufacture of goods in the United States. This is one of the reasons manufacturing has been moving outside the country, creating unemployment in America.

The changes recommended in this book are only for the healthcare industry and not for other sectors of the economy. In other areas of the economy, such as manufacturing, free enterprise and capitalistic system are working quite well and do not need change.

If you want to characterize the system of healthcare recommended in this book as social medicine, then *yes* this *social medicine* can save our *capitalistic economy* by making it more efficient.

12. To bring down medical costs, could we use group practices that pay doctors a salary but keep rest of the system unchanged?

President Obama has praised clinics such as Mayo Clinic and Cleveland Clinic, which pay doctors a salary and also have a reputation for delivering high quality healthcare. Canadians also often use these clinics when they travel to the United States for their healthcare needs. President Obama has stated that these clinics can serve as role models for the delivery of healthcare in America. A similar idea has been expressed by health policy expert Dr Arnold Relman (41).

While President Obama as well as Dr. Relman have offered their sincere opinions that are worthy of respect, neither one of them has explained why this approach would bring down healthcare costs at a national level.

While requiring doctors to work in group practices on a salary basis is yet another way to deliver healthcare, it is not enough. Even though Mayo Clinic and Cleveland Clinic are doing an excellent job, they still use the same type of unsafe medicine based mostly on drugs and surgeries that is being practiced elsewhere in the country. Being private institutions they still have the need to maximize their profits.

The system would also not be as simple as the one suggested in this book. When it comes to healthcare, simplicity is a virtue. It makes very little sense to burden sick people with decisions about finances, or treatments choices about their healthcare plan. When one is sick one must be able to walk into one of the healthcare facilities and get needed treatment without worrying about having to make decisions from a multitude of options, many of which the patient does not understand.

13. Some say that one reason why healthcare costs keep going up is because more technology keeps on developing. Even if we change the system, could costs go up due to development of new technologies?

In free markets, the type of technology that gets developed and adopted is the technology that brings efficiency and thus brings down the costs. Or the new technology provides more capability, but at a reasonable cost. Our healthcare system offers opposite incentives; only those treatments and medical technologies are being developed that make money for the providers thus raising the costs.

Once the incentives for the providers are changed, the focus will shift from developing technology that makes money for the providers to developing technology that is more beneficial to the patients. Only those technologies will be developed that are more cost effective. Thus, even with new technologies, the costs will not rise but might fall.

14. Can HMOs Offer a Solution to our Healthcare Problems?

At first, it might appear that if fee-for-service medicine is at the root of all our healthcare problems, then Health Maintenance Organizations (HMOs) might offer a solution.

However, the country has had experience with the HMOs. They have not been popular with patients. While a rational patient would be on guard whether he or she is being over-medicated or under-medicated, in practice most patients only complain when they are being under-medicated. Because HMOs are private for-profit entities who can make bigger profits by denying treatments, most people did not trust them. For the same reasons, they are not likely to trust them in the future.

15. You said that by switching to a British-like system we can reduce the national expenditures on healthcare to about 40 percent of what we are spending now. But, won't we have to offer our doctors much higher salaries than the British doctors are currently being paid? Won't these salaries have to be comparable to what American doctors are currently making in private practice? If so, won't this increase the cost of the system?

In the earlier days of the switch, we would need to pay American doctors higher salaries than those being paid to

British Doctors to attract them into the new system. But, the savings that will result by changing the system will also be *due to the change in the practice of the type of medicine that would follow from the changed system.* Savings will occur due to fewer hospitalizations and less use of expensive drugs. Doctors' incomes are only one of the factors in the overall healthcare costs. Other factors are hospital costs and the cost of drugs. In the long run, doctors' salaries will be fixed by the demand for doctors versus the number of medical graduates available to fill that demand.

When doctors are not in private practice, they would be free from the influence of drug representatives who want to push more expensive patented drugs. More non-drug approaches using much safer natural substances would be used for medicine.

Another form of saving would come from hospitals that now would be government owned. Hospital costs form a major portion of any medical bill. Experience shows that government-owned hospitals in other countries cost only a fraction of what the private hospitals in America cost, as shown in Chapter 1.

If we have trouble moving the American doctors into the new system, we must not forget that there are experienced doctors who currently practice in Europe or other developing countries, but want to migrate to the United States. Currently, they are being prevented from migrating because of the immigration restrictions. Immigration restrictions for doctors can be loosened during the period we are changing our system.

The sooner we can change the system and provide free coverage to everyone, the better...Such a system can lift the worry about health thus adding to the quality of life of Americans. Many of us work hard all our lives and still die destitute and are robbed of all our dignity toward the end of our lives just because of the faulty healthcare system. Citizens of our great country deserve better.

EPILOG

I hope that this book has answered the basic question posed in its title. Namely, why healthcare in America is so expensive? In short, it is the combination of two elements in our system. First, is the practice of paying doctors on a fee-for-service basis. Second is the use of third-party private insurance to pay for these services.

The quality of medical care is decreasing because we are not making payments for health but for doctors' services, which might or might not improve a patient's health. The costs are accelerating because the money patients are spending is mostly not theirs but the insurance companies'.

If we paid our doctors on a fee-for-service basis and patients had to pay with their own money, the system would not be so expensive, although, it would still not be a great system. However, people would be more judicious with their money and demand more value for it. However, healing would not be based solely on expensive surgeries or potentially harmful drugs.

Healing would be based on more judicious use of natural substances and knowledge of the human body. Emphasis would be on prevention and maintenance of health rather than on medical intervention. Medical intervention would be used only in rare cases, such as accidental injuries or other health emergencies.

But, we are not recommending such a system. With all its benefits, this type of system would be very burdensome on the sick. Fee-for-service method of payment, does work with some degree of success in some areas of the economy such as auto mechanics, where people spend from their own pockets, and therefore demand results for the service they pay for.

Our present healthcare system is more than fair to doctors who get paid for every service they render whether their service is beneficial to the patient or not. It is unfair to the patients (or their insurance companies) who must pay for every effort whether or not it helps them.

If we knew how to precisely quantify health, and knew precisely how much the service of a doctor has added to our health in the short and long run, we could conceivably design a system that pays doctors fairly even if we used insurance to pay them. Unfortunately, we do not know how to quantify health; therefore, this type of system is difficult to conceive.

This leaves us with only one alternative: to pay the doctors on a salary basis. While it is not a perfect method of payment and does not provide any additional financial incentives beyond the satisfaction that comes from healing the sick, *it is better than providing the wrong incentives.*

Although, both the cost and quality are issues with our system, the problem of cost is more obvious, because costs can be easily measured.

Our well-equipped hospitals and expensive doctors well trained in surgeries can sometimes give the impression to the uninitiated that our system must be good. Only when the outcomes in our system are compared with the outcomes in other countries does the quality issue become apparent.

But cost is an important issue and is the one that has been emphasized throughout this book. Many of the current problems in our society, such as the increasing number of bankruptcies resulting from unpaid and grossly inflated medical bills and lack of adequate medical coverage for significant number of people are the result of the high cost. At the national level, the high cost of healthcare is making it difficult forAmerican businesses to compete effectively in the international markets.

But the good news is that these *same* factors in our system that are responsible for medicine's high cost are also responsible for its lowered quality. By changing the system, we can improve on *both*. We do not have to spend more money to get better healthcare. We can improve quality by spending less.

Fortunately, we have working models of systems in which this has been done. United Kingdom provides an excellent example. It provides complete coverage to all its citizens at 40 percent the cost per person of what the United States spends.

This is good news for the United States because the U.S. government already spends nearly 40 percent of all healthcare dollars spent in the country. This means that by changing the system, the U.S. government can provide free universal coverage to all its citizens without raising taxes. This step would provide coverage for everyone, and *make our businesses more competitive internationally.* The *long-term outlook on Social Security will also improve.*

The only disadvantage of a totally free system such as that in United Kingdom is that we might have longer waiting periods for non-emergency surgeries. Although such waiting periods are inevitable in any totally free system, those who do not mind waiting can get all their healthcare for free. Those, who do not want to wait, can buy supplemental insurance. But even for those who choose to buy supplemental insurance, the cost of additional insurance would be less than what they are paying now. Because of a parallel free system, the costs of medicine to those who want to pay for it would be much less.

In addition to cost savings, the new system will also encourage prevention. Instead of emphasizing more medical intervention, healthcare providers can emphasize prevention without the fear of loss of income.

The sooner we can change the system and provide free coverage to everyone, the better. In addition to the more quantifiable benefits of lowered costs, such a system can lift the worry about health thus adding to the quality of life of Americans. It should make society more productive by allowing citizens to focus on more productive pursuits rather than having to worry about their health coverage. In our society, many of us work hard all our lives and still die destitute and are robbed of all our dignity toward the end of our lives just because of the faulty healthcare system. Citizens of our great country deserve better.

WORKS CITED

1. **Davis, Karen, Ph.D. et al.** *Mirror, Mirror on the Wall.* The Commonwealth Fund, 2010 Update.

2. **Centers for Medicare and Medicaid Services.** [Online] [Cited: 5 26, 2014.] http://www.cms.gov/Research-Statistics-Data-and-Systems/Statistics-Trends-and-Reports/NationalHealthExpendData/NationalHealthAccountsHistorical.html.

3. **Buhner, Stephen Harrod.** *Herbal Antibiotics, : Natural Alternatives for Treating Drug-resistant Bacteria.* 2nd Edition. Storey Publishing, LLC, 2012. p. 480 pages. ISBN-13: 978-1603429870.

4. **McKenna, John.** *Natural Alternatives to Antibiotics.* Avery, 1998. p. 208. ISBN-13: 978-0895298393.

5. **Pollack, Andrews.** Doctors Denounce Cancer Drug Prices of $100,000 a Year. *The New York Times.* April 5, 2013.

6. www.goodrx.com. [Online] [Cited: May 28, 2014.] http://www.goodrx.com/avastin?gclid=COSO7NTZzb4CFWsO OgodrgcAig..

7. **Mandal, Dr Ananya, MD.** Avastin (Bevacizumab) Price. May 28, 2014, News Medical.

8. **Henderson, Bill.** *Cancer-Free: Your Guide to Gentle, Non-toxic Healing.* Booklocker.com, Inc., 2007. ISBN-13: 978-1601451835.

9. **Servan-Schreiber, David.** *Anticancer: A New Way of Life.* Viking Adult; New edition, 2009. ISBN-13: 978-0670021642.

10. **Francis, Raymond.** *Never Fear Cancer Again: How to Prevent and Reverse Cancer* 1st edition, 2011. ISBN-13: 978-0757315503.

11. **Gerson, Charlotte.** *The Gerson Therapy: The Proven Nutritional Program for Cancer and Other Illnesses.* Kensington; Reissue edition, 2001. ISBN-13: 978-1575666280.

12. **Evans, R.** Supplier-Induced Demand: Some Emperical Evidence and Implications. *The Economics of Health and Medical Care.* 1974.

13. **Office of Inspector General.** *Financial Interests Between Healthcare Arrangements Between Physicians and Healthcare Businesses.* Washington, D.C. : Department of Health and Human Services, 1989.

14. **Hillman, B et al.** Frequency and Cost of Diagnostic Imaging in Office Practices: A comparison of self-referring and Radiology-referring Physicians. *New England Journal of Medicine.* 1990.

15. **Roemer, M.I.** Bed supply and hospital utilization: a natural experiment. *Hospitals.* 1961.

16. Certificate of need. *Wikipedia.* [Online] [Cited: October 19, 2014.] http://en.wikipedia.org/wiki/Certificate_of_need.

17. **Rubinstein J, F Aloka, G S Abela** Statin therapy decreases myocardial function as evaluated via strain imaging. *Clinical Cardiology.* December 2009.

18. **Blaylock, Russell L.** *Excitotoxins: The Taste That Kills.* Health Press (NM), 1996. ISBN-13: 978-0929173252.

19. Drug Company Used Ghostwriters to Write Work Bylined by Academics, Documents Show. [Online] ProPublica. [Cited: April 27, 2014.] http://www.propublica.org/blog/item/drug-company-used-ghostwriters-to-write-work-bylined-by-academics-documents.

20. **Wilson, Duff.** Drug Maker Hired Writing Company for Doctors' Book, Documents Say. *New York Times.* November 29, 2010.

21. **Angell, Marcia.** *The Truth About the Drug Companies: How They Deceive Us and What to Do About It.* Random House Trade Paperbacks, August 2, 2005. ISBN-13: 978-0375760945.

22. **Whitaker, Robert.** *Anatomy of an Epidemic: Magic Bullets, Psychiatric Drugs, and the Astonishing Rise of Mental Illness in America.* Broadway Books, August 2, 2011. ISBN-13: 978-0307452429.

23. **Dumit, Joseph.** *Drugs for Life: How Pharmaceutical Companies Define Our Health.* Duke University Press Books, September 3, 2012. ISBN-13: 978-0822348719.

24. **Lind, James.** *A Treatise on the Scurvy.* 1753.

25. **Cohen, Suzy.** *Diabetes Without Drugs: The 5-Step Program to Control Blood Sugar Naturally and Prevent*

Diabetes Complications. Rodale Books, November 9, 2010 ISBN-13: 978-1605296753.

26. **Friedman, Milton.** How to Cure Healthcare. *Hoover Digest.* July 30, 2001.

27. **Kohn, Linda T et al.** *To Err is Human: Building a Safer Health System.* Washington, DC : National Academies Press, 2000. ISBN: 0-309-51563-7.

28. **Committee on Quality of Health Care in America.** *Crossing the Quality Chasm: A New Health System.* Washington, DC : National Academies Press, 2001. ISBN: 0-309-51193-3.

29. **Han Y Y, J A Carcillo, S T Venkataraman, R S Clark, R S Watson, T C Nguyen, H Bayir, R A Orr** Unexpected increased mortality after implementation of a commercially sold computerized physician order entry system. *Pediatrics.* December 2005.

30. **Evans, Dwight C. , W. Paul Nichol, and Jonathan B. Perlin.** *Effect of the implementation of an enterprise-wide Electronic Health Record on productivity in the Veterans Health Administration.* Issue 02, April 2006, Health Economics, Policy and Law, Volume 1, pp 163-169.

31. **Groopman, Jerome and Pamela Hartzband.** Obama's $80 Billion Exaggeration. *The Wall Street Journal.* March 12, 2009.

32. *Canadian Institute for health Information.* https://www.cihi.ca/en Retrieved October 30, 2012.

33. **Makary, Marty.** *Unaccountable: What Hospitals Won't Tell You and How Transparency Can Revolutionize Health Care.* Bloomsbury Press. ISBN-13: 978-1608198382.

34. **Davis, Karen et al.** *Mirror Mirror on the Wall 2014 Update.* New York : The Commonwealth Fund , 2014.

35. **Tamkins, Theresa.** Medical bills prompt more than 60 percent of U.S. Bankruptcies. *CNNhealth.com.* [Online] June 5, 2009. [Cited: June 18, 2014.] http://www.cnn.com/2009/HEALTH/06/05/bankruptcy.medical. bills/index.html?_s=PM:HEALTH.

36. **Evidence-Based Medicine Working Group.** Evidence-based medicine. A new approach to teaching the practice of medicine. *JAMA The Journal of the American Medical Association.* November 4, 1992.

37. **Hughes, G B** Evidence-based medicine in health care reform. *Otolaryngol Head Neck Surg.* October 2011.

38. **Siefe, Charles.** Is Drug Research Trustworthy? *Scientific American.* December 3, 2012.

39. **Taylor, Renee.** *Hunza Health - Secrets for Long Life and Happiness.* Prentice Hall, Inc. ASIN: B000K6S272.

40. **Price, Weston A.** *Nutrition and Physical Degeneration.* Price-Pottenger Nutrition Foundation . ISBN-13: 978-0916764203.

41. **Relman, Arnold.** *A Second Opinion: A Plan for Universal Coverage Serving Patients Over Profit.* Century Foundation Books (PublicAffairs), 2010. p. 240. ISBN-13: 978-1586488062.

42. 1951 Food, Drug, and Cosmetics Act Amendments. *Durham-Humphrey Amendment, Public Law 82-215.* Cited in the end notes.

43. **Starr, Paul.** *The Social Transformation of American Medicine: The rise of a sovereign profession and the making of a vast industry.* Basic Books, 1984. ISBN-13:978-0465079353. Cited in the end notes.

44. **Chlebowski RT, Anderson GL, Gass M, et al.** Estrogen Plus Progestin and Breast Cancer Incidence and Mortality in Post-menopausal Women. *JAMA. 2010; 304 (15):1684-1692. doi:10.1001/jama.2010.1500.* Cited in the end notes.

45. **Davis, Devra.** *The Secret History of the War on Cancer.* Basic Books, February 24, 2009. ISBN-13: 978- 0465015689. Cited in the end notes.

46. **Fries, James F.** Aging, Natural Death, and the Compression of Morbidity. *New England Journal of Medicine.* 1980, Vol. 303, 3, pp. 130-35. Cited in the end notes.

47. New York state medical malpractice coverage premiums. *Excellus.* [Online] [Cited: November 10, 2014.] https://www.excellusbcbs.com/wps/wcm/connect/b7cdbf66-dd6b-4fb0-9612-47112e93c9f7/Med+Malpractice+FS+2014-EX+FINAL.pdf?MOD=AJPERES&CACHEID=b7cdbf66-dd6b-4fb0-9612-47112e93c9f7. Cited in the end notes.

48. **Ablin, Richard J.** The Great Prostate Mistake. *The New York Times.* March 9, 2010. Cited in the end notes.

49. The Texas Economy. *Texas Healthcare Costs.* [Online] [Cited: November 1, 2014.] http://thetexaseconomy.org/healthcare/costs/articles/article.ph p?name=healthcare. Cited in the end notes.

50. **Wennberg, John E.** *Tracking Medicine: A Researcher's Quest to Understand Health Care.* 1st edition. Oxford University Press, 2010. ISBN-13: 978-0199731787. Cited in the end notes.

51. **Kennedy, Edward.** *In Critical Condition: The Crisis in America's Health Care.* Simon & Schuster, 1972. ISBN-13: 978-0671213145. Cited in the end notes.

BIBLIOGRAPHY

Abramson, John. *Overdosed America: The Broken Promise of American Medicine.* Harper Perennial, 2008.

Angell, Marcia. *The Truth About the Drug Companies: How They Deceive Us and What to Do About It.* Random House Trade Paperbacks, 2005.

Birch, Joseph T. *Cystic Fibrosis ~ Alternative Treatments.* CreateSpace Independent Publishing Platform, 2013.

Blaylock, Russell L. *Excitotoxins: The Taste That Kills.* Health Press (NM), 1996.

Blum, Susan. *The Immune System Recovery Plan: A Doctor's 4-Step Program to Treat Autoimmune Disease.* Scribner, 2013.

Boodman, Sandra, "Misdiagnosis is more common that drug errors or wrong site surgery," *Washington Post.* May 6, 2013. Retrieved from https://www.washingtonpost.com/national/health-science/misdiagnosis-is-more-common-than-drug-errors-or-wrong-site-surgery/2013/05/03/5d71a374-9af4-11e2-a941-a19bce7af755_story.html (Retrieved on November 13, 2015).

Bowles, Jeff T. *Why Is There No Multiple Sclerosis at the Equator? How Brazilian Doctors Are Curing MS with High-Dose D3.* CreateSpace Independent Publishing Platform, 2013.

Brawley, Otis Webb and Paul Goldberg. *How We Do Harm: A Doctor Breaks Ranks about Being Sick in America.* St. Martin's Griffin, 2012.

Brownlee, Shannon. *Overtreated: Why Too Much Medicine Is Making Us Sicker and Poorer.* Bloomsbury USA, 2008.

Buhner, Stephen Harrod. *Herbal Antibiotics, : Natural Alternatives for Treating Drug-Resistant Bacteria,* 2nd Edition. Storey Publishing, LLC, 2012.

Carter, James P. *Racketeering in Medicine: The Suppression of Alternatives.* Hampton Roads Publishing Compan, 1992.

Centers for Medicaid Services (CMS). http://www.cms.gov/Research-Statistics-Data-and-Systems/Statistics-Trends-and-Reports/NationalHealthExpendData/NationalHealthAccountsHistorical.html

Cohen, Suzy. *Diabetes Without Drugs: The 5-Step Program to Control Blood Sugar Naturally and Prevent Diabetes Complications.* Rodale Books, 2010.

Commonwealth Fund. "Mirror, Mirror on the Wall, 2014 Update: How the U.S. Health Care System Compares Internationally," June 16, 2014. Retrieved from http://www.commonwealthfund.org/publications/fund.org/ publications/fund-reports/2014/jun/mirror-mirror.

Davis, Devra. *The Secret History of the War on Cancer.* Basic Books. 2009.

Desaulniers, Veronique. *Heal Breast Cancer Naturally: 7 Essential Steps to Beating Breast Cancer.* TCKPublishing.com, 2014.

Epstein, Samuel S. *The Politics of Cancer Revisited* . East Ridge Press, 1998.

Francis, Raymond. *Never Fear Cancer Again: How to Prevent and Reverse Cancer.* HCI; 2011.

Gerson, Charlotte. *The Gerson Therapy: The Proven Nutritional Program for Cancer and Other Illnesses.* Kensington; Reissue edition, 2001.

Griffin, G. Edward. *World Without Cancer: The Story of Vitamin B17.* American Media, 2013.

Groopman, Jerome. *How Doctors Think.* Mariner Books, 2008.

Haley, Daniel. *Politics in Healing: The Suppression and Manipulation of American Medicine.* Potomac Valley Press, 2000.

Henderson, Bill. *Cancer-Free: Your Guide to Gentle, Nontoxic Healing.* Booklocker.com, Inc., 2007.

Hyman, Mark *The Blood Sugar Solution: The UltraHealthy Program for Losing Weight, Preventing Disease, and Feeling Great Now!* Little, Brown and Company, 2014.

Hyman, Mark *Ultraprevention.* Atria Books, 2005.

Kennedy, Edward. *In Critical Condition: The Crisis in America's Health Care.* Simon & Schuster, 1972.

McDougall, John A. *The McDougall Program for a Healthy Heart: A Life-Saving Approach to Preventing and Treating Heart Disease.* Dutton, 1996.

McKenna, John. *Natural Alternatives to Antibiotics.* Avery, 1998.

Morrison, Ian. "Health Care Costs and Choices in the Last Years of Life." March 30, 2015. Hospitals and Health Networks (HHN). Retrieved from http://www.hhnmag.com/articles/3656-health-care-costs-and-choices-in-the-last-years-of-life

Myers, Amy M.D. *The Autoimmune Solution: Prevent and Reverse the Full Spectrum of Inflammatory Symptoms and Diseases* . HarperOne, 2015.

National Foundation for Transplants. "How Much Does a Transplant Cost?" September 28, 2010. Retrieved from http://www.transplants.org/faq/how-much-does-transplant-cost.

Organization for Economic Cooperation and Development. http://www.oecd-ilibrary.org/.

Price, Weston A. *Nutrition and Physical Degeneration: A Comparison of Primitive and Modern Diets and their Effects*. Price-Pottenger Nutrition Foundation , (originally published 1939).

Swenson, Nicole. *Multiple Sclerosis: How I Reversed My Chronic Autoimmune Symptoms By Making Simple Changes To The Way I Eat*. Talent Writers, 2014.

Taylor, Renee. *Hunza Health - Secrets for Long Life and Happiness*. Prentice Hall, Inc., 1978.

Thomas, Lewis. *The Youngest Science*. Penguin Books; Reprint edition , 1995.

Wennberg, John E. *Tracking Medicine: A Researcher's Quest to Understand Health Care.* Oxford University Press, 2010.

Endnotes

[1] Even though the *Affordable Care Act* is a step in the right direction toward universal coverage, it falls short of its goal as will be discussed in Chapter 5.

[2] For the data provided by the Centers for Medicaid Services (CMS) see http://www.cms.gov/Research-Statistics-Data-and-Systems/Statistics-Trends-and-Reports/NationalHealthExpendData/NationalHealthAccountsHistorical.htm Last retrieved November 2, 2014.

[3] Certainly some people claim that the American system is the best in the world, but there are no studies supporting these claims.

[4] Health: Key Tables from the Organization of Economic Cooperation and Development (OECD) at http://www.oecd-ilibrary.org/ - Retrieved on October 15, 2014.
and the following publication:
OECD (2013), Health at a Glance 2013: OECD Indicators, OECD Publishing, Paris.

[5] See "Mirror, Mirror on the Wall, 2014 Update: How the U.S. Health Care System Compares Internationally," a Report by the Commonwealth Fund, June 16, 2014. Retrieved from http://www.commonwealthfund.org/publications/fund.org/ publications/fund-reports/2014/jun/mirror-mirror

[6] On end-of-life care, see, for example, Ian Morrison, "Health Care Costs and Choices in the Last Years of Life." March 30, 2015. Hospitals and Health Networks (HHN). Retrieved from http://www.hhnmag.com/articles/3656-health-care-costs-and-choices-in-the-last-years-of-life

[7] All data presented in Chapter 1, is taken from ' 2010 Comparative Price Report' by International Federation of Health Plans.

[8] According to many experts this number is too low because not all doctors report all their errors due to fear of malpractice suits.

[9] For a comprehensive discussion of medical errors that routinely occur in American hospitals, see Ref (27).

[10] As of this writing, Nexium has become available for over-the-counter purchase.

[11] Patent for Lipitor also recently expired. The prices quoted here were prices in 2010.

[12] The price of Lipitor quoted in France is the price of a generic substitute Tahor.

[13] In addition to the systems mentioned on page 38, there is also the VA system that covers a small number of Americans, but does not use the 'two pillars' for payments to providers. Since very few Americans are covered under this system, it does not have a significant impact on American Healthcare prices.

[14] Needless to say, the medical profession loves the system.

[15] The healthcare industry has a vested interest in setting very high standards for health. Most people find it impossible to meet these standards. For a discussion of what health parameters (such as blood pressure and so forth) are considered normal today versus what was considered normal a few years ago, see the book by Marcia Angell (21).

[16] Household income source from Henry J. Kaiser Family Foundation, updated October 9, 2015, retrieved from http://kff.org/other/state-indicator/median-annual-income/.

[17] I am not suggesting that we keep the fee-for-service payments for doctors but abolish insurance. The observation is only meant to point out how payment systems can affect medical prices and practice.

[18] The graph is drawn in nominal dollars. But costs have been increasing even when measured in real dollars. For example, another significant measure of this growth is the total healthcare costs as a percentage of GDP. In1960, we spent only 5 percent of GDP on healthcare. In 2012 this ratio was 17.2 percent.

[19] Insurance companies refer to demand for unnecessary utilization of medical care as "moral hazard."

[20] Some readers might object to my reference to patients as "consumers," but in a market-based system for delivery of medicine, the words are synonymous.

[21] The extent of prescription drugs prescribed is mammoth. The percentage of persons using at least one prescription drug in the past thirty days: 48.7% (2009-2012); the percent of persons using three or more prescription drugs in the past thirty days: 21.8% (2009-2012); and the percent of persons using five or more prescription drugs in the past thirty days: 10.7% (2009-2012). Source: Centers for Disease Control. Data table for Figure 20. "Prescription drug use in the past 30 days, by number of drugs taken and age: United States, 1988–1994 through 2007–2010." Retrieved from http://www.cdc.gov/nchs/hus/contents2013.htm#fig20. In general the trend has been towards prescribing more drugs.

[22] 1951 Food, Drug, and Cosmetics Act Amendments. See Ref (42).

[23] As a perfect example, I once remember listening to a radio show host who said that if a drug did not have serious side effects, he did not want to take it because he *knew* it won't be effective! He never explained how he reached that conclusion.

[24] In 2012, government expenditures represented about 40 percent of the total national dollars spent on healthcare. This ratio has been nearly constant for the last several years. See Reference (2).

[25] The role of monitoring agency such as the Food and Drug Administration (FDA) is not being questioned. We can continue to have an agency such as the FDA to oversee the effectiveness and safety of drugs. But, there is no reason why a doctor's prescription should be required for their purchase, once the drug has been approved by the FDA. After all, we allow unrestricted purchase of fire arms by all citizens even though they are much more dangerous than drugs.

[26] The advent of private health insurance dates back to 1929, the year of the stock market crash that marked the beginning of the great depression. The first noteworthy insurance plan was offered by the Baylor University Hospital. To generate income in these economically depressed times, it offered insurance to public school teachers at the cost of 50 cents a month to provide coverage of up to 21 days of hospital stay. The idea took off. Very soon many such plans proliferated in the market. By 1937 there were 26 such plans with 600,000 enrollees. It also led to the establishment of all popular Blue Cross Hospital Insurance. For more details on the subject see (43). By 1950s employer based health insurance was commonplace. Since then the system has had a major impact on many aspects of medical practice. It is also worthwhile noting that the system of payment

for healthcare using private insurance has its origins *in the needs of the medical providers* (in this case Baylor University Hospital) *rather than the needs of the patients.* That is why the system originated in the economically depressed times. It was the industry's need to sell more medicine that changed the system. To this day, the medical industry tries to overmedicate the general public for profit. The evidence of this assertion will be provided in the next chapter where well known concepts such as 'Romers' Law' and 'Supplier Induced Demand' (12) are discussed.

[27] This type of reform has been recommended by many politicians and many Americans believe it to be the ultimate solution to healthcare reform. As we will see, this reform will be an improvement over the present system but is not the ultimate solution.

[28] Although because of its monopoly powers as a payer, Canada can better control the price of a given service that a doctor performs, when it comes to *the number of services* that a doctor will perform, the Canadian government has lesser control. The doctors still have a lot of leeway in how many tests to order or how many procedures to perform on a given patient.

[29] For other reasons why Canada has lower costs than the U.S see Chapter 5 under the section. 'Single-payer system.'

[30] Some other examples show that government comes to the rescue of people when the business model becomes unviable for the private insurers. For example, in some areas in Florida that are prone to hurricanes, government insurance is the only insurance that people buy. Also, after the September 11, 2001 terrorist attacks, private insurance companies have refused to insure property against terrorist attacks. However, the federal government has stepped in to fill in this gap.

[31] For population over the age of sixty-five years, the American Medicare system is like the Canadian system except that in the United States, the hospitals are private, whereas in Canada hospitals have very different structure. Even the private hospitals in Canada are strictly controlled by provincial governments. Their operations are often managed either by community boards or volunteer organizations. They can essentially be characterized as government entities, and are quite inexpensive compared to American Hospitals.

[32] A single payer with monopoly powers of a payer is in a better position to negotiate prices with the healthcare providers.

[33] Except infrequently during routine physicals or 'well-woman' visits.

[34] Malpractice suits are higher in those specialities that practice more risky medicine. In 2013-14 the standard malpractice premium for a general practitioner in Long Island Counties of New York was only$37,877 but a general surgeon paid more than three times that amount at$141,608 (47).

[35] The original law passed by New York is sometimes referred to as the Metcalf- McCloskey Act.

[36] A collection of studies related to this topic are available at http://www.dartmouthatlas.org/. Retrieved 1-4-2014. See also (50).

[37] A study conducted in December 2009 by J. Rubinstein of the Cardiology Division, Department of Medicine, Michigan State University showed that statin therapy *decreases* myocardial function. See reference (17) for more details.

[38] For a more detailed discussion on this topic, see the excellent book by Dr. Marcia Angell, which discusses this topic in more detail. See reference (21).

[39] For example, a paper published in JAMA in October 20, 2010 by R. T. Chlebowski, et al. concluded that therapy with estrogen plus progestin was associated with a greater incidence of breast cancer. See Reference (44).

[40] Routine tests are often used by providers as a first step to get patients into their offices, in order to sell them more medicine.

[41] For example, regular mammograms expose the body to harmful radiation and can thus be the cause of the cancer that they are supposed to prevent. Use of PSA testing for determining prostate health has been criticized by the very researcher who played a key role in developing the test (48). Tonsillectomies were once very popular and were routinely performed on children. Their worth is now debated and they are not performed as frequently. They can be harmful because they remove the tonsils that are a part of the immune system and can thus weaken the immune system.

[42] One group of people with the longest lifespan in the world is the Hunza. These people live long lives without much medical intervention Ref (39).

[43] The Dr. Weston Price Foundation website at http://www.westonaprice.org/ provides information about dental care and nutrition.

[44] Nearly all drugs are toxic substances that must first be detoxified by the liver. The byproducts of this detoxification process then must be eliminated through the kidneys. Thus, nearly all drugs stress out your liver and kidneys in addition to having other side effects.

[45] For example, earlier in this chapter, we pointed out how statin drugs often prescribed to help in the heart function can actually harm the heart·

[46] CAT scans can have radiation equivalent to hundreds of X-rays. For a good discussion about radiation levels in various medical procedures, see reference (45).

[47] It is disconcerting to observe that American lawmakers want to solve the problem of high drug prices in America by allowing re-importation through Canada rather than by fixing the system at home.

[48] Many companies such as AETNA or Cigna sell other forms of insurance in addition to health insurance. They are not part of healthcare industry.
[49] Despite potential problems, some people have already experienced the benefits of EMRs. A friend told me that before EMRs he had to wait for weeks for test results needed in connection with his stepdaughter's surgery and then he had to hand-carry paper copies to the doctor. Now, the test results are available online within hours.
[50] This might not be true of preventive office visits or routine checkups.
[51] See GAO-08-474R Health Savings Accounts, Retrieved from http://www.gao.gov/new.items/d08474r.pdf
[52] For example, see http://www.medicareforall.org/pages/Home (Retrieved on November 9, 2014).
[53] Quite possibly, the advocates of this system see the duplication of the Canadian system in the United States.
[54] Under our current system, healthcare providers are the biggest beneficiaries of the system and as such are also the biggest voice opposed to any changes to the system.
[55] Many major insurance companies in the United States, such as Cigna and Aetna, provide many other insurance products in addition to healthcare. Such a solution would, therefore, be less disruptive to such companies.
[56] In the United States, a similar strategy has been used to curb costs. Some states require special permission in the form of a 'Certificate of Need' before hospitals or other healthcare facilities can be built. I am not a fan of this strategy for controlling costs for reasons mentioned in Chapter 4.
[57] No matter what system of delivering healthcare we settle on, the *system should be simple*. It is a burden on the sick to require them to make complex healthcare decisions when they are already sick. In the design of healthcare system, *simplicity is a virtue in itself.*
[58] The insurance industry is not even a part of the medical industry. Some of the same companies such as Aetna and Cigna that sell health insurance also sell auto and home insurance. Those who recommend reforming the insurance industry are looking for a solution in the wrong place.
[59] Reforming the insurance industry for its own sake is a worthy goal, but tinkering with the insurance industry to bring down the underlying medical costs significantly is an unreasonable expectation.
[60] https://www.cms.gov/Research-Statistics-Data-and-Systems/Statistics-Trends-and-

Reports/NationalHealthExpendData/NationalHealthAccountsHistorical.htm
l Retrieved October 8, 2015.

[61] The vision of the healthcare system expressed here already exists in the Great Britain. Senator Ted Kennedy in his 1972 book also outlined a similar vision of this healthcare system. See reference (51).

[62] In Chapter 8 we will discuss why even double blind studies are not adequate.

[63] Most Brits are very proud of their system. It has consistently been rated number one among select industrialized nations (34)

[64] Even in our present system, it can take a long time to set up an appointment to see a good doctor especially if you are a new patient in a big city.

[65] Americans are not as egalitarian as the Canadians. Therefore, it would be better for our society to allow people to buy private insurance and get ahead of other people in line and get treatment from a private doctor if they can afford it. This type of system works quite well in England.

[66] In a salaried system, doctors still have the incentive to be good doctors because they are being watched by the management. Any feedback provided to their superiors can affect their salaries and promotions.

[67] Some readers might feel that we cannot achieve the same level of savings in the United States as the British because we will have to offer American doctors higher salaries. True, but despite having to pay higher salaries than the British, we will still lower healthcare costs because the new system will function under changed incentives. Under the new system, doctors will have no incentive to deliver too much medicine or expensive medicine.

[68] Even though doctors insist that medical education is more expensive than other professions, this is not accurate. Currently, most medical schools, law schools, and many graduate and undergraduate schools (such as Harvard or George Washington University in Washington, DC) charge the same yearly tuition of about $50,000 per year to all. Though medical education takes a year longer than law school, it takes on average less time than getting a Ph.D. in the sciences or arts.

[69] The National Health Service Corps will repay loans for people who agree to work in under-served, often low-income areas. The corps' Loan Repayment Program offers up to $60,000 in tax-free loan repayment in exchange for two years of full-time service, or four years of part-time. There are also other programs that offer similar inducements to doctors to get them to practice in these areas.

[70] Period from 1929 to 1950s marked the growth period for the use of insurance to pay for healthcare.

[71] How Much Does a Transplant Cost? National Foundation for Transplants. September 28, 2010. Retrieved from http://www.transplants.org/faq/how-much-does-transplant-cost.

[72] Alternative medicine has also saved lives, in many cases when modern medicine failed.

[73] The possibility of people living long lives and dying without generating end-of-life medical costs has been studied and is referred to in the medical literature as "Compression of Morbidity." Dr. James Fries, professor of medicine at Stanford University School of Medicine, first put forward this hypothesis in 1980. For reference to his original paper see (46).

[74] In our present system, the threat of medical lawsuits serves as an antidote to excessive and unsafe medicine.

[75] Boodman, Sandra, "Misdiagnosis is more common than drug errors or wrong site surgery," *Washington Post*. May 6, 2013. Retrieved from https://www.washingtonpost.com/national/health-science/misdiagnosis-is-more-common-than-drug-errors-or-wrong-site-surgery/2013/05/03/5d71a374-9af4-11e2-a941-a19bce7af755_story.htmlRetrieved on November 13, 2015).

[76] This is not to say that our legal system does not have its faults. It is just a comparison with other countries. For example, in countries such as India and in certain Latin American countries, court cases can languish in courts for many years before decisions are made.

[77] It is worth noting that about two-thirds of the states in the United States already have some sort of limits on awards in tort cases.

[78] From 2005 to 2009, healthcare spending in Texas rose more than 36 percent. See (49).

www.ingramcontent.com/pod-product-compliance
Lightning Source LLC
Chambersburg PA
CBHW051446170526

45166CB00001B/132